PRINCIPLES
of
MOVEMENT

PRINCIPLES *of* MOVEMENT

Brent D. Anderson, PT, PhD, OCS, NCPT
Assistant Professor
Doctor of Physical Therapy Program
University of St. Augustine for Health Sciences

Founder/CEO
Polestar Education, LLC
Miami, Florida

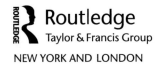

Routledge
Taylor & Francis Group

NEW YORK AND LONDON

First published in 2024 by SLACK Incorporated

Published 2024 by Routledge
605 Third Avenue, New York, NY 10017
4 Park Square, Milton Park, Abingdon, Oxon OX14 4RN

Routledge is an imprint of the Taylor & Francis Group, an informa business

© 2024 Taylor & Francis Group

Brent D. Anderson is the owner and founder of Polestar Education, LLC.

Library of Congress Cataloging-in-Publication Data

Names: Anderson, Brent (Physical therapist), author.
Title: Principles of movement / Brent Anderson.
Description: Thorofare, NJ : SLACK Incorporated, [2023] | Includes
   bibliographical references and index.
Identifiers: LCCN 2023022097 (print) | ISBN 9781630914684 (hardcover)
Subjects: MESH: Movement--physiology | Exercise Movement Techniques |
   Exercise Therapy | Kinesiology, Applied--methods | BISAC: MEDICAL /
Allied Health Services / Physical Therapy | MEDICAL / Sports Medicine
Classification: LCC RM725 (print) | NLM WE 103 | DDC
   615.8/2--dc23/eng/20230727
LC record available at https://lccn.loc.gov/2023022097

ISBN: 9781630914684 (hbk)
ISBN: 9781003525912 (ebk)

DOI: 10.4324/9781003525912

DEDICATION

I dedicate this book in memory of my father, Delbert L. Anderson.
Thank you for your continual support and raising me to finish the job.

CONTENTS

ACKNOWLEDGMENTS

The cliché "it takes a village" is as true as it gets in the completion of this book. There are so many people who have inspired me to achieve this goal in my professional life. I would like to start by thanking my mentors, Dr. Nancy N. Byl from the University of California San Francisco and Dr. Carol M. Davis from the University of Miami, who have always encouraged me to maximize my potential.

I would also like to thank my family and my colleagues at Polestar Education, LLC. My wife, Lizette, thank you, my love, for your daily support of my dreams and your patience through the difficult times. My mom, Fern, thank you for your unconditional support and for transcribing 16 hours of video presentation into hundreds of pages to begin the book. My daughter, Alina Anderson, thank you for being such a talented artist and helping me in the last stages of compiling the first draft of the book. Thank you for drawing the abstract art pieces at the beginning of every chapter. My daughter, Nichole Anderson, thank you for your support and choice to help run and direct the curriculum in Polestar so that I could complete the book. Your insight and contributions to the final edits are invaluable. My son, Gabriel Anderson, thank you for taking an executive role in the company and always encouraging me to finish. My daughter-in-law, Martha Miller, thank you for your excellent proofreading skills, one of your many talents.

Kelly Anderson, chief illustrator and Pilates teacher, made it possible to depict an artistic and scientific depiction of movement and movement science. Thank you! My executive assistant and chief of staff, Elizabeth Jimenez, always motivated me and helped me make time in my busy life to finish the book. Thank you for playing such a major role in the final stages of preparing all the content for submission. My all-time editor and education partner for almost 30 years, Shelly Power, thank you. I could not have done this without your help. Your continual prompting to make the content accessible and meaningful at the same time is priceless. My lifelong friend and graphic designer, Gary Bentz, thank you for your invaluable help with the final illustrations in the book and your consistent encouragement to finish this project. Thank you to Andreina Santaella, Polestar chief operating officer, colleague, and driving force to always finish what one starts. My colleague, Beth Kaplanek, thank you for your help starting the formal process of writing and laying out the book. Your encouragement and example were so valuable. My colleague, Christi Idavoy, thank you for being my resource for energy and my yoga inspiration. My colleague and dear friend of more than 25 years, Angela Crowley, thank you for providing your expertise in Gyrotonic Expansion System, Feldenkrais Method, and Pilates. My colleague and fellow visionary on health and what a health-based practice should look like, Staffan Elgelid, thank you for your guidance on the book and your contribution to the section on Feldenkrais. My colleague from Israel, Hadar Schwartz, thank you for keeping me accurate with my interpretation of the research and for being my first reader of the book in its rawest form. My colleague, friend, and licensee in Spain, Juan Nieto, thank you for consulting with me on this book and always making me aware of current, pertinent, and meaningful research. My dear friends Dav Cohen, Lise Stolze, and Alastair Greetham, thank you for being instrumental in the development of the original Polestar Principles of Movement course more than 25 years ago. My first Pilates teacher and partner for more than a decade, Elizabeth Larkam, thank you for helping me to see the power of movement in rehabilitation. Your impact in the medical community is most impressive.

I would be remiss if I did not thank God for the abundance of opportunity provided to me to grow and be surrounded by so many amazing people in my life. I am grateful for the peace, love, and hope that have always been shown to me.

ABOUT THE AUTHOR

Brent D. Anderson, PT, PhD, OCS, NCPT is a licensed physical therapist and orthopedic certified specialist who has practiced physical therapy for more than 30 years. In 1989, he received his degree in physical therapy from the University of California San Francisco and completed his studies in the Pilates method with Elizabeth Larkam at the Center for Sports Medicine at Saint Francis Memorial Hospital in San Francisco, California. He continued to learn from first- and second-generation Pilates teachers, including Eve Gentry, Carola Trier, Ron Fletcher, Romana Kryzanowska, Kathy Grant, Lolita San Miguel, Mary Bowen, Jean-Claude West, and Alan Herdman.

After graduating, Dr. Anderson moved back to his hometown, Sacramento, California, and started practicing physical therapy; he embarked on a journey filled with continual learning and practice. Several years later, the then–Chair of the Department of Physical Therapy and Rehabilitation Science at the University of California San Francisco, Dr. Nancy N. Byl, PT, MPH, PhD, FAPTA, encouraged him to seek his doctoral degree.

In 1997, Dr. Anderson moved to Miami to pursue his doctoral degree at the University of Miami. It was there that he met his lifelong professional friend and mentor, Dr. Carol M. Davis, DPT, EdD, MS, FAPTA. His doctoral dissertation focused on chronic low back pain and the comparison of active vs passive intervention, as well as the comparison of behavioral vs physical measures and their ability to predict outcomes. In 2005, Dr. Anderson completed his doctorate in physical therapy at the University of Miami.

Dr. Anderson's professional studies did not stop there. His professional growth continued with years of intense manual therapy training and practice combined with more than 30 years of dance medicine and Pilates education, myofascial studies with Dr. Davis, and personal investigation and practice of energy medicine and meditation. His unique skill set has allowed him to create an exciting and holistic approach to health and well-being.

Dr. Anderson is the founder and CEO of Polestar, one of the leading Pilates education companies in the world. At the time of printing, Polestar has provided Pilates education and teacher training in more than 60 countries and in 15 languages since 1992. Dr. Anderson was involved in the development of the Pilates Method Alliance (PMA) Pilates Certification Program and the PMA Certification Examination and served on the PMA (now the National Pilates Certification Program) Certification Commission.

Dr. Anderson has become a renowned lecturer at national and international symposia and consults with physical therapists, dance companies, universities, and other educational bodies throughout the world. He is a leading authority in performing arts medicine, Pilates for rehabilitation, pain management through movement, and spine health. He is currently an assistant professor at the University of St. Augustine for Health Sciences, and serves on the board of directors for the School of the Arts for Boys Academy and Bgood.org, a community-empowering organization. He has served as president of the Performing Arts Special Interest Group of the orthopaedic section of the American Physical Therapy Association and is the past chairman of the board of directors for Shake-a-Leg Miami.

PREFACE

We all move, but when was the last time you thought about what you were doing? The complex orchestra of thoughts, reflexes, desires, bones, muscles, tendons, nerves, fascia, and skin contribute to our spontaneous ability to move through life. If you move, appreciate movement, teach movement, enhance movement, or restore movement, then this book is for you. I have been intrigued with understanding how we as humans learn to move from a very early age. One of my first impactful professional encounters occurred at the California Physical Therapy Association Annual Conference where Dr. Helen Hislop, the director of the University of Southern California, gave the keynote address. This is when she introduced the concept of "pathokinesiology" to me as a definition of physical therapy. I have never looked back and have embraced her definition of physical therapy ever since 1989. I am a pathokinesiologist; any trauma, disease, or mental impairment that interferes with the ability to move is my specialty. I learned early on that the restoration of movement is the focal point in my career, which meant that I would need to learn everything I could about movement and how pathology affects movement. This book is a compilation of my studies, practice, experiences, and struggles pertaining to Principles of Movement. The objectives of this textbook are to enhance the ability of the practitioner to assess normal movement, assess movement that has been impaired by pathology, and design unique movement interventions for everyone with whom we work. This book includes strategies, tools, and algorithms for movement practitioners that will significantly improve the odds of reaching the desired outcomes.

The longer we live, move, and experience life, the more our "biography" layers over our neuromyofascial system with patterns of movement that reflect not only our experiences but our thoughts and feelings about those experiences.

Meister Eckhart, a philosopher from the 1300's, has said,

"There is a place in the soul that neither time nor space nor no created thing can touch."

John O'Donohue, the great Irish poet, responded,

"What that means is that your identity is not equivalent to your biography, and that there is a place in you where you have never been wounded, where there is still a sureness in you, where there's a seamlessness in you, and where there is a confidence and tranquility in you. And I think the intention of prayer and spirituality and love is, now and again, to visit that inner kind of sanctuary."[1]

This book reflects one clinician scholar's work devoted to help movement educators to access our awareness of that place inside our patients that has never been wounded and bring it forward to assist in the return to pain-free, integrated movement grounded in pure joy.

I first met Brent Anderson when he made his way into my office at the University of Miami in Coral Gables in the mid-1990s. He was excited to talk with me because, it turns out, he made his way to us as a doctoral student knowing that one of the faculty members had an interest in what we then called "complementary therapies." That would be me, gladly. I was beginning to publish more about the merits of a holistic view of our patients and the promising outcomes of therapies that were grounded in subtle energy to complement our traditional treatments.

Before making his way to Miami, Brent had been active as a physical therapist in Pilates methodology and practice for several years in California and had a goal to investigate the scientific foundations behind what he felt was the premier effectiveness of this modality that could not be grounded yet in scientific terms. He saw Pilates as a complementary holistic therapy, ideally positioned to assist physical therapists and other rehabilitation professionals in movement education. With its emphasis on spiral motion and full body involvement in movement, assistance, and resistance, from specific whole-body cueing and highly calibrated spring mechanisms, people really enjoyed moving and exercising. His commitment to investigating Pilates and the science that made it so effective was very exciting to witness.

We move forward now to 2023. Brent completed his PhD long ago, and the 30th anniversary of his multinational corporation, Polestar, was recently celebrated. Polestar practitioners can be found in more than 60 countries around the world. Their qualification as a Polestar practitioner is a highly valued achievement awarded after many hours of study and practice in one of the most rigorous Pilates curricula available in the world.

And so, along with the 30th anniversary of Polestar, emerges Brent's book, *Principles of Movement*, that you hold in your hands, based on his years of experience, as well as his dissertation and ongoing research into the scientific foundations of the "magic" behind the Pilates work. As you work your way through this text, you'll recognize how Brent has collated and perfected his understanding of movement science and Pilates practice into five basic Principles of Movement that are supported by the scientific foundations of movement from evolving literature over the years.

These five principles—**breath, mobility, alignment, control,** and **movement integration**—coalesce into an evaluation and treatment approach, supported by strong science, and are incorporated into an assessment and treatment tool that Brent makes available to the reader of this book, regardless of background in Pilates practice.

Indeed, this book is not just written for Pilates practitioners. It represents an example of a valued contribution to the new, cutting-edge science and art of movement education for all professionals, written to train the eye and heart of the practitioner to meet each patient with individual awareness, curiosity, and evaluation and teaching skills.

Early in his practice, Brent discovered that movement is affected by all "systems of being" and he incorporates an understanding of the latest research in the scientific foundations of movement: anatomy, physiology, biomechanics, kinesiology, motor learning, psychology, sociology, and bioenergetics. Although most readers will have a basic understanding of these areas of study, this will be an introduction to bioenergetics for many. Bioenergetics represents the growing science of subtle energy, which serves as the foundation for the holistic cohesion of all these influences on human movement into a congruent, integrated, self-actualized whole, fostering homeostasis and balance through vibrational flow throughout the entire living fascial web.

Individual perceptions, both known and unknown, influence how we feel and how we move. For example, for many decades the International Association for the Study of Pain, composed of clinicians and researchers working together to understand sources and mechanisms of pain, accepted this definition of pain:

"An unpleasant sensory and emotional experience associated with actual or potential tissue damage or described in terms of such damage."

In 2018, the International Association for the Study of Pain formed the 14-member multinational presidential task force charged to examine that definition of pain and to recommend whether it should be retained or changed. Indeed, the definition was then tweaked, in a subtle, but oh-so-powerful way.

The new definition reads as follows:

"Pain is an unpleasant sensory and emotional experience associated with *or resembling that associated with* actual or potential tissue damage."[2]

This advisory panel had realized the wisdom that pain is highly individualized and based on a patient's perception of past experiences located deep in the body and the nervous system. This definition gives agency to a patient's story in a way that moves the symptom of pain subtly away from measures that record solely objective quantification and incorporates qualification, description funded by individual perception. Evaluation instruments had to be altered to incorporate this enlightened definition.

In this same spirit, this book takes us from the written world of anatomy and physiology, functional anatomy, and kinesiology into the world of the perceptual lived reality of "embodiment." What does it mean to feel your anatomy, your physiology in the way you move? And how do those individual feelings, known and unknown, affect the way we move?

Brent suggests that:

"The better we understand the diversity in pain interpretation, neuromuscular responses, historical perspective of pain and the individual, and physiological and psychological adaptation, we can start to see how complex and beautiful movement science is. Qualitative and conscious movement training will continue to become a big part of the future of motor learning especially in therapeutic interventions. By enhancing awareness and being able to improve our use of external and internal feedback tools, we can improve the alignment between perception and reality … I use the word reality in a framework to understand what the real needs of the client are, not a fabricated one that is applied in a blanket strategy. **How do we discover the individual in front of us and truly understand their needs from the movement practitioner's perspective?** … The question for us should be: How will we choose **to influence our client's belief system?**

- Will it be through creating positive movement experiences without pain?
- Will it be through graded load exercises that progress toward a more functional load desired by the client?
- Will it be through a restoration of mobility that alleviates stress in other parts of the body and allows pain-free movement?
- Will it be through regaining motor control of the body through meaningful external and internal feedback strategies, including imagery, tactile and verbal queuing, and internal reflection?"

A deeper awareness of what the practitioner is seeing is brought to the focus approximating the lived experience of "integrated wholeness." Freedom of movement and pain-free movement are at the heart of what is desired.

Intelligence that is centered in the head is extremely limited. We all feel emotion but not all of us are aware of how subconscious emotion, which is ever present in the deeper body, is expressed in our movements. Brent teaches the reader to bring a learned eye, applying these principles in a holistic way, to suggest subtle changes in position, alignment, focus of power, and control. He teaches how to discern if interrupted efficiency, alignment, and power are due to structural pathology or impaired holding and movement strategies collected over time.

But before all this, he starts with meaningful interview. He asks the patient, "What do you believe you should be able to participate in right now? Do you believe you are currently able to participate in this activity at the level you desire? And if not, what do you believe is challenging or preventing you from participating at the level you desire?" And then he listens for their responses and adjusts his evaluation and treatment protocol incorporating his 5 principles accordingly, ensuring meaningful personalization. What a different approach to examination and evaluation for exercise.

This is a book that assists all movement educators to improve their scientific knowledge and their assessment, treatment, and teaching skills. I am thrilled to see it published.

—*Carol M. Davis, DPT, EdD, MS, FAPTA*
Professor Emerita
Department of Physical Therapy
University of Miami Miller School of Medicine
Clinician, Myofascial Release Physical Therapist
Coral Gables, Florida

REFERENCES

1. Tippett K. On Being – Interview with John O'Donohue. The Inner Landscape of Beauty. https://onbeing.org/programs/john-odonohue-the-inner-landscape-of-beauty/
2. IASP newsletter. July 16, 2020. IASP announces a revised definition of pain. https://www.iasp-pain.org/publications/iasp-news/iasp-announces-revised-definition-of-pain/

INTRODUCTION

As movement practitioners, how well do we truly understand the many factors that influence the quality of movement? I have spent my career as a physical therapist and Pilates teacher exploring various methodologies to have a better understanding of the integration of movement assessment and movement facilitation. My passion for movement, healing, science, and human behavior has driven this lifelong work with the goal of helping doctors, nurses, therapists, trainers, coaches, teachers, athletes, dancers, and anyone who is interested in optimizing movement achieve a new movement potential by embodying the Principles of Movement.

Helen Hislop, PhD, PT, the director of the University of Southern California's physical therapy program for 23 years, made a comment about physical therapists being *pathokinesiologists*. Dr. Hislop wanted physical therapists to understand that the profession should be focusing on restoring movement to individuals who were experiencing movement-impairing diseases, congenital anomalies, traumas, and any other physical or psychological limitation. For this to be true, the practitioner must be an expert in the science of movement and the effects that disease and injury have on the effectiveness and efficiency of functional movement. The tone of this book is truly written for the pathokinesiologist and the performance kinesiologist in all of us. The focus of this text is designed to facilitate problem solving and movement enhancement through a deeper understanding of movement principles that are applicable to Pilates, yoga, and Gyrotonic Expansion System teachers; athletic trainers; exercise physiologists; massage therapists; physical therapists; chiropractors; osteopaths; orthopedic physicians; and anyone passionate about human movement. This text relies on the teachings of many great pioneers in movement education, biomechanics, motor control, and the amazing methods of yoga, Pilates, Gyrotonic Expansion System, Feldenkrais Method, dance, and martial arts.

Many of the great movement pioneers could have been labeled as *pathokinesiologists* according to their teachings and treatment of clients with movement pathologies. They worked with individuals who had postural and movement deviations and created exercises to help balance the imbalances, often through an exploration of movement efficiency.

The role of a pathokinesiologist is to be the expert in how pathology affects movement. With that being said, I would like to introduce and coin the phrase "performance kinesiologist." The role of the performance kinesiologist is to be the expert in how the quality of movement can affect individuals from a post-rehabilitation state all the way to high levels of function and performance. Both require a deep understanding of qualitative movement that can only come through the practice of conscientious movement. The ability to incorporate conscientious movement into our own movement practice will significantly enhance our effectiveness in the restoration of function and enhancement of performance for our clients. In this book, I refer to both the pathokinesiologist and the performance kinesiologist as the *movement practitioner*.

This book introduces and explains how the application of movement principles can enhance the practitioner's ability to facilitate qualitative movement safely, timely, and effectively with their clients. These movement principles have been a work in progress for many years with the help of many great minds from many fields of movement science. We first introduced the Principles of Movement as a course more than 30 years ago in the Polestar curriculum. We created the course to bring a science-based foundation to Pilates. The Polestar Principles of Movement can serve as a foundation for all movement practices. This book shows you how to incorporate the principles into your work and improve your efficiency by changing your approach to working with clients whether your emphasis is rehabilitation, postrehabilitation, wellness, or performance. Each principle discussed in this book is supported by evidence-based research from multiple scientific fields. The importance of the anatomical, physiological, biomechanical, kinesiological, psychological, and energetic systems of the human being as they pertain to movement are included in this book.

This book is designed to be used as a textbook for courses revolving around movement science. I expect it to be used in both vocational and professional education. It is ideal for dance, physical education, recreational therapy, physical therapy, occupational therapy, and exercise science programs. The primary learning objectives of this textbook are as follows:

1. Observe and assess functional movement using the Principles of Movement.
2. Observe and assess movement impairments caused by genetics, habits, trauma, or pathology using the Principles of Movement.
3. Use the Polestar Assessment Tool and integrate it with the International Classification of Functioning, Disability and Health.
4. Design movement-based interventions to improve performance and restore function using the Principles of Movement.

This text is also designed as a resource for movement professionals. It contains a depth of information that I hope will continue to support practitioners as they mature in the fields of rehabilitation, postrehabilitation, conditioning, and performance.

All readers and users of this book should practice within their scope as defined by their local government, professional organizations, and/or places of employment. Scope of practice laws and guidelines are in place to protect the public. While I was in my doctoral studies, there is one thing that I learned, "The more I know, the more I know I don't know." There is often a false sense of confidence that accompanies ignorance when the following can be said—"The less I know, the more I think I know." I ask that all readers and users of this material use it safely and within their appropriate scope of practice.

I hope that you and all users of this book will frequently return to its pages. Continued study combined with your own evolving movement awareness will lead you down the path of becoming a master mover and teacher of movement.

For additional information and resources, please visit principlesofmovementbook.com.

PHOTO CREDITS

The following pages have illustrations by Alina Anderson: pp. 24, 56, 98, 124, 150

The following figures were created by Chris Frisina: 4-1, 4-8, 4-24, 4-26, 4-27, 4-30, 4-33, 5-9

The following figures were created by Gary Bentz: 3-1, 3-5, 5-3, 6-1, 6-2B, 6-8, 6-9, 6-10, 7-4, 7-5, 8-1, 8-2

The following figures were created by Jafar Fallahi: 3-11, 5-5, 5-7, 5-8, 5-10

The following figures were illustrated by Kelly Anderson: 3-2, 3-3, 3-4, 3-7, 3-9, 3-13, 3-14, 3-15, 3-16, 3-17, 3-18, 3-21, 3-22, 4-2, 4-3, 4-4, 4-5, 4-6, 4-7, 4-8, 4-9, 4-10, 4-11, 4-12, 4-13, 4-15, 4-21, 4-22, 4-23, 4-25, 4-31, 4-32, 4-33, 4-34, 4-35, 4-36, 4-37, 4-38, 4-39, 4-40, 4-41, 5-1, 5-2, 5-6, 5-8, 6-2B

The following figures were created by Polestar Education, LLC: 1-1, 1-2, 3-6, 3-10, 3-23, 5-2, 6-3, 6-4, 6-5, 6-6, 6-7, 8-2

The following figure was created by Sara Radosavljevic: 4-20

The following figure was created by Sharon Ellis: 3-19, 3-20

INTRODUCTION TO PRINCIPLES OF MOVEMENT

"WHOLE BODY COMMITMENT IS MENTAL AND PHYSICAL DISCIPLINE, A WORK ETHIC, AN ATTITUDE TOWARD ONESELF, AND ASSUMING A LIFESTYLE THAT IS NECESSARY TO ACHIEVE WHOLE BODY HEALTH."

Joseph Pilates

CHAPTER OBJECTIVES

1 Identify the basic sciences that can relate to movement.

2 Understand how the basic sciences apply to movement science.

3 Explain how the basic sciences influence movement.

4 Integrate basic sciences into the application of each of the Principles of Movement.

KEY TERMS

- Alignment
- Arthrokinematics
- Bioenergetics
- Biomechanics
- Breath
- Congruence
- Control
- External feedback
- Functional anatomy
- Internal feedback
- Kinesiology
- Mobility
- Motor control
- Motor learning
- Movement integration
- Osteokinematics
- Physiology
- Pilates
- Psychology
- Sociology
- Yoga

After graduating from physical therapy school and completing my initial Pilates training, I practiced the Pilates movements a few hours a day, almost every day of the week, for more than a year. It was a powerful learning experience for me. I observed how the Pilates movements affected each of my body's systems. I was able to observe how alignment, tension, and load affected different tissues in the neuromuscular and skeletal systems. What appeared to be restrictions based on old beliefs of muscle tightness or stiff joints were replaced with images of suppleness, elasticity, and coordination. I realized that my own restrictions were much more responsive to strategy and awareness training than the structural restriction model I had been taught. This model, which was built on passive manipulation and

stretching followed by isolated strength training of muscles, was slowly being replaced by a model of awareness, motor control, and strategy. My observations continued to expand as I imagined the effect of movement on the digestive, circulatory, and respiratory systems. Imagine how a mobile spine could affect motility, blood flow, and air exchange. Years later, as I was studying how movement of the physical body can influence our psychological, emotional, and energetic systems, it became very apparent to me that movement affected all systems of being, and if I were to be an expert in movement, I would have to understand what I refer to as the *scientific foundations of movement*—anatomy, physiology, biomechanics, kinesiology, motor learning, psychology, sociology, and bioenergetics.

Anderson BD.
Principles of Movement (pp 2-12).
© 2024 Taylor & Francis Group.

I was very privileged to have met and observed many of the first-generation Pilates teachers. Although their exercises and sequencing varied from one to another, they shared common underlying principles, such as breath, flow, precision, and alignment. Many of these principles were difficult to quantify. As a young physical therapist, I wanted to explain the advantages of the Pilates method to my profession; to do this, Pilates needed evidence-based research.

I was asked by colleagues in the therapy profession to provide scientific evidence supporting Pilates as a therapeutic modality. I wanted to legitimize Pilates in the scientific world and create a set of movement principles that would be supported by science. Pilates teachers were also interested in working with populations with spinal pathologies, neurologic conditions, amputations, and a whole host of other diseases and traumas. We needed to identify the magic behind the Pilates work to be able to modify it and make it accessible to everyone. By following sound movement principles, the practitioners could make the method client-centric vs exercise-centric.

I investigated, with a team of friends in the profession, the original repertoire of Joseph Pilates and his guiding principles and work from many leaders in the movement science field to develop the Polestar Principles of Movement. Over the past 25 years, these principles have evolved into breath, mobility, alignment, control, and movement integration. Each of these principles was specifically thought through as global or holistic Principles of Movement supported by scientific foundations of movement. Our interpretation was based on our mixed experiences with other disciplines, including yoga, Gyrotonic Expansion System, martial arts, dance, Feldenkrais Method, the Franklin Method, manual therapies, neurolinguistic programming, and energetic medicine studies. The primary goal was to understand the many factors that influence movement and then discover how to guide our clients toward a healthier movement experience, and as Joseph Pilates stated, "return to life."

Each of the Principles of Movement is organized into 2 sections. The first section consists of "science you need to know," and the second section is the application of the movement principle. The first section of each chapter presents the movement sciences, or as I refer to in this book, the 5 scientific foundations of movement. The second section of each chapter consists of teaching skills that are incorporated into each principle, including but not limited to communication, touch, emotional intelligence, movement acquisition, and motor learning. They are accompanied by a practical application through suggestions of bony landmark identification, imagery, tactile cueing, and basic communication skills. These combined skills enhance the teacher's ability to apply the Principles of Movement to their teaching. Lastly, each chapter includes key terms and open-ended questions to increase the book's effectiveness and enhance learning.

FUNCTIONAL ANATOMY/ PHYSIOLOGY

Have you ever thought about a movement as basic as walking? Most of us only think of the goal or the task from the outside (eg, "I need to get from here to there"). Could you imagine having to tell every muscle when to fire and what percentage of recruitment is needed, or worse yet, having to remember which muscle fires first, second, and so on? To find the balance between understanding our muscle anatomy and what we will refer to as *functional anatomy*, we must think of movement as a collective orchestration. The brain does not know one muscle from the other; it knows movement. This does not reduce the need to know our muscle anatomy; rather, it enables us to think of it in a functional manner. The first scientific foundation is human anatomy and physiology as it pertains to movement. Functional anatomy addresses the relationship between structures. Take our example of walking. The myofascial system provides the appropriate amount of tension to efficiently bear the vertical load of gravity as we locomote one leg at a time. This is different than just identifying the origin, insertion, and function of an isolated muscle. The vastus medialis by itself cannot maintain the leg or body in an upright stance, but when integrated with all the other necessary muscles and fascia and preceded by a command from the central nervous system to move, the orchestra begins; some muscles provide stiffness, whereas others accelerate and decelerate motion. In this book, I will assume that you already know your basic musculoskeletal anatomy and that you can progress into the anatomical relationships as they pertain to synergistic and functional movement organization and the disruption to the movement system secondary to pathology. The better the practitioner or teacher understands functional anatomy, the easier it becomes to move and teach movement with efficiency and accuracy.

I have had the opportunity to work with many dancers over the years, and one of the most common problems is their lack of understanding of where the hip joint is and how the femur articulates with the pelvis. Historically, classical ballet has taught the need for turnout (ie, external rotation). It is an aesthetic line that in classical ballet is a must, and it is also something that many dancers do not naturally possess. If the dancer does not understand exactly where their hip joint is or how to turn out from

there or simply does not have that range of motion, then they will get their turnout from somewhere else, such as the knee, ankle, or foot. None of these structures are meant to take the place of true hip external rotation. When dance teachers and choreographers understand hip joint anatomy, biomechanics, and movement strategy, then their teaching will respect the dancers' structure, and dancers will be more likely to work safely within their movement limits, resulting in improved performance and a decreased likelihood of overuse injuries. When we understand that the actual hip joint is very close to the central axis and not where the greater trochanter is, then weight shifting and hip external rotation become significantly easier and more efficient.[1] It is crucial that all movement practitioners become very knowledgeable with the anatomy of the skeletal, musculotendinous, articulating, and fascial structures.

I mentioned my study of Pilates through the lens of the different body systems. As I deepened this practice, for the first time I could understand how the Pilates roll up exercise (Figure 1-1) could improve the flow of body fluids, oxygen transport through better circulation, cellular nutrition, and the removal of waste, hence enhancing homeostasis. Ancient well-being practices such as yoga teach us the importance of knowing the anatomy and the physiological systems as they are part of whole body movement.

BOX 1-1: ANATOMY IMAGERY EXPERIENCE 1

Stand up so that your weight is equal on both legs, and imagine you are being suspended from the ceiling by a heavy elastic band. Allow your skeleton to dangle as if you are a Halloween decoration. Further imagine the wind blowing your skeleton from behind. Feel your body sway forward and backward; notice where tension increases and decreases. Find the point where you experience the least amount of tension throughout your body. Can you identify your central axis? Can you feel any imbalances in the external tissues as you sway back and forth? Can you imagine your pelvis articulating with your femur as your body sways? Record your findings, including the subtleties you experience; try again in a few days, and see if you observe something different.

BOX 1-2: ANATOMY IMAGERY EXPERIENCE 2

Using anatomical landmarks can make it much easier to explore successful movement than cueing or using voluntary muscle contractions. In this experience, from a standing posture, begin to forward bend; imagine your right lung moving over your liver and your left lung moving over your stomach and spleen. Repeat the same activity; however, this time imagine you are articulating each segment of the thoracic and lumbar spine. Is there a difference? Did one feel easier for you to accomplish the task of forward bending? Try other movements that focus on moving through or around other bony landmarks or organs. Record your experience.

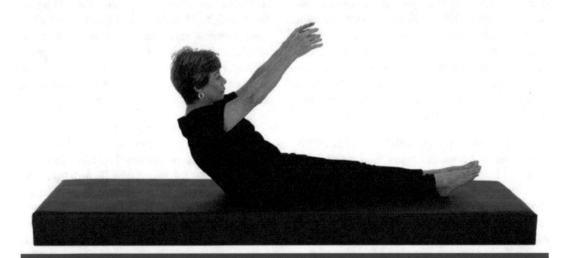

Figure 1-1. The roll up exercise.

BIOMECHANICS

Biomechanics, the study of the mechanical laws relating to the movement or structure of the human body, is one of my favorite movement sciences. If we truly understand the nature of movement in the joints and the forces that are required to move the skeleton through space, we can begin to appreciate how the nervous system and myofascial system interact to produce movement. I find it fascinating to learn what our biomechanical movement potential is vs what we manifest in our daily activities. Every joint is composed of at least 2 bones that form a union and together create movement in varying planes depending on the nature of the joint. Joints are acted on by external forces such as gravity or momentum and can also be acted on internally by the myofascial contractions. Each "true" joint, consisting of a capsule, synovium, and cartilage, has at least 2 articulating surfaces. In synovial and cartilaginous joints, the articulating surface decreases friction and provides directional movement. When the joint surfaces fit together well, we say they are congruent.

Congruent articulation involves both osteokinematics (ie, movement of the bones) and arthrokinematics (ie, movement of the joints). Osteokinematics refers to the physiological motion of the joint, such as flexion, extension, abduction, adduction, pronation, supination, eversion, inversion, and rotation. Arthrokinematics is synonymous with the accessory motion of the joint. Another term for this used by Eric Franklin is *bone rhythms*.[1] Arthrokinematics takes into consideration the nature of the joint and its movement properties. For example, the knee is a bicondylar joint with accessory motions, including spin, glide, and spiral. I like to compare movement in the joint to opening the lid of a jar. The lid and the jar must move in opposite directions to open or close. If they move in the same direction, there is no movement in that joint, and forces can be transferred to other joints to compensate for the lack of movement in the desired joints. If you can create images or ideas that match the natural arthrokinematics in the body, the resulting movement will be more efficient and powerful. Think about a novice movement strategy as having over-recruitment, poor arthrokinematic awareness,

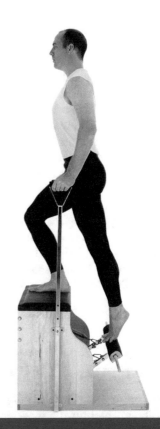

Figure 1-2. A forward lunge on the chair.

BOX 1-3

I once treated a professional basketball player who had multiple surgeries on his left knee, which was his jumping leg. His last surgery was successful, resulting in what appeared to be a very stable and strong left knee; yet, his biggest complaint was his loss of elasticity and the inability to jump. After evaluating his knee biomechanics, I realized that through all his prior physical therapy, he had never been assessed or treated to restore the accessory joint mechanics of the knee postsurgery. However, he was strong, and the ligaments appeared to be very stable. I focused his treatment on the arthrokinematics (bone rhythms) of the left knee—spin, glide, and spiral motions— while performing an assisted lunge on a piece of Pilates equipment known as the chair. Within minutes, he expressed that he felt a significant return of his natural elasticity that he had been missing since his last surgery. The next day, he commented that he was able to jump high enough to get his elbow over the rim, something I could only dream about. I am always impressed when what appears to be a structural restriction (ie, a loss of ankle dorsiflexion or knee flexion) is instead a strategic restriction that resolves almost immediately once correct biomechanical strategies have been restored (Figure 1-2).

and decreased power compared with a skilled movement strategy in which you can imagine sound biomechanics, increased power, and decreased energy expenditure. The science of biomechanics and arthrokinematics enables the movement teacher to access a much deeper comprehension of how and where movement occurs. It helps identify what the ideal is or what should be happening beneath the surface. When restrictions occur, whether structural or strategic, there is often a loss of congruence, which leads to compensatory patterns and often pathology.[2,3] Likewise, when the student is free from restrictions and moves with good strategies, they will experience a significant increase in movement efficiency and theoretically minimize the risk of injury.

MOTOR CONTROL AND MOTOR LEARNING

Motor control and motor learning sciences are also fundamental for the movement practitioner who wants to successfully facilitate movement in their clients. The scientific models of motor learning and motor control help us understand the acquisition and control of movement in the body and in the environment; they also help us to comprehend multiple factors that influence movement. As we better understand these models of motor control and motor learning, we become better problem solvers. Humans learn to do things through practice. External feedback from the environment or a teacher helps facilitate the successful completion of the desired task. Taking it one step further, we encourage clients to explore their internal feedback, which helps to solidify the learning process. Think of a child learning to write. The formation of the letters is choppy and unorganized, but with practice, it becomes smooth and coordinated. In the beginning, you had to focus all your attention while writing your name; now you do it without any conscious thought. Understanding how humans learn and acquire movement empowers a movement practitioner's ability to implement a large array of tools and strategies to enhance the learning process. An understanding of motor learning also helps us know how to set up the most effective practice sessions for our clients. There are many great minds in the field of motor control who I will be leaning on to help us understand the most effective ways to facilitate spontaneous and efficient movement.

PSYCHOSOCIAL SCIENCES

Psychology and behavioral sciences have been successfully incorporated into the movement sciences over the past number of decades. It is the relationship of how belief, hope, and perception impact movement and how movement impacts the psyche. Self-perception has great bearing on how one performs movement. Current research has indicated that the perception of a successful movement experience can decrease pain, overcome fear, and significantly improve the quality of movement.[4-7] Fear of movement as it relates to the anticipation of pain is known as *fear avoidance* and is thought to be a major predictor of poor functional outcomes. *Self-efficacy*, which was defined by Albert Bandura, is a term used to describe one's perception of their ability. Functional outcome measures, such as the Oswestry Disability Index and the Roland-Morris Questionnaire, measure an individual's perception of how their back pain interferes with their perceived ability to work.

The literature supports a correlation between perception and ability.[4,5,8-13] If you believe you will get better from your injury, you probably will. The reverse is also true; if you believe you will not get better, you probably will not, no matter how strong, flexible, or coordinated you are. Anecdotally, students of Pilates, Gyrotonic Expansion System, yoga, Feldenkrais Method, tai chi, and other movement disciplines report feelings of increased calmness, happiness, and peacefulness; decreased stress; and better social interactions. How do successful movement experiences affect our psychological and emotional

BOX 1-4

While teaching the concept of body, mind, and spirit some years ago to a group of students, I shared a story of a woman whose physical symptoms were a direct result of her religious belief. She originally presented with a 2-week history of back pain. Her imaging tests came back negative for any mechanical pathology in her low back. Two more weeks went by with physical therapy and Pilates, and there was still no change. We were both frustrated with her lack of improvement, and because I could not see any structural or physiological reason for the pain to persist, I asked her what she thought was causing her low back pain. Her response surprised me as she threw up her hands in the air and said, "God is punishing me." I allowed her to continue to tell her story, and it turned out she was having an affair with her husband's coworker. Being a very religious woman, she believed this was a cardinal sin and that God's punishment was being manifested as low back pain. I relayed to her that she had 3 options to resolve her dilemma and her back pain: she could go through the repentance process within her belief model, she could change her belief into one of free love and sex, or she could continue to have low back pain. She responded almost immediately that her back no longer hurt; when I asked again what hurt, she replied that it was her heart that hurt. The reason why I share this very personal story is to convey the message that our mind and spirit can influence our physical health just like our physical health can influence our mind and spirit. This was Joseph Pilates' underlying principle—a healthy body is the first step toward happiness.

well-being? In his philosophy of Contrology, Joseph Pilates emphasized that the attitude toward oneself was critical to achieving whole body health.[14] The design of the Pilates equipment provides an assistive environment for the mover. If taught correctly, Pilates can create positive movement experiences that result in a paradigm shift of one's belief in their ability to move.[4]

"WHOLE BODY COMMITMENT IS MENTAL AND PHYSICAL DISCIPLINE, A WORK ETHIC, AN ATTITUDE TOWARD ONESELF, AND ASSUMING A LIFESTYLE THAT IS NECESSARY TO ACHIEVE WHOLE BODY HEALTH."
—JOSEPH PILATES[14]

BIOENERGETICS

In his book *Energy Medicine in Therapeutics and Human Performance*, James Oschman defined bioenergetics as the "field of the future" in which there is an intersection between biology and energy or "the study of the flow and transformation of energy in and between living organisms and their environment."[15] The link between biology and energy is vast and includes biochemistry; cellular communications; biophysics; and neurobiology, including the role of photons, energy psychology, and more. These topics are all researched by the National Center for Complementary and Integrative Health (NCCIH), the federal government's lead agency for scientific research on complementary and integrative health approaches. Complementary approaches can be classified by their primary therapeutic input (how the therapy is taken in or delivered), which may be:

1. Nutritional (eg, special diets, dietary supplements, herbs, probiotics)
2. Psychological (eg, mindfulness)
3. Physical (eg, massage, spinal manipulation)
4. Combinations, such as psychological and physical (eg, yoga, tai chi, acupuncture, dance or art therapies) or psychological and nutritional (eg, mindful eating)[15]

Why is it important to understand the relationship between nutrition, mindfulness, touch, and energy fields as a movement practitioner? How do disturbances in the body's systems impact whole body health? To better answer this relationship between energy and movement, we can refer to ancient and modern movement forms that incorporate the connection between body, mind, and spirit and how they influence illness and wellness.

The practice of yoga is more than 5000 years old. Hatha yoga (ie, yoga of physical forces) is what most people in the Western world relate to as yoga, including Ashtanga, Iyengar, Bikram, and many more. The 8 limbs of yoga have physical exercises known as *asanas*, breath control known as *pranayama*, and other practices that serve as a prescription for moral and ethical conduct and self-discipline; they direct attention toward one's health, and they help us to acknowledge the spiritual aspects of our nature. According to Simon Borg-Olivier, hatha yoga is, in essence, a type of tantric yoga with 4 physical stages: cleansing, physical exercise, energy control, and breath control.[16] This book is not about the practice of yoga but will draw from its historical perspective as it applies to the Principles of Movement.

Joseph Pilates had similarly linked philosophies of hygiene, control, breath, and balance in life.[14] There is little literature demonstrating the integration of meditation into the original practice of Joseph Pilates, known as Contrology, but the Pilates sequences are often thought by many to be a movement meditation and thus able to produce positive psychological and emotional responses.[17,18] Joseph Pilates wrote the following: "Contrology is complete coordination of body, mind, and spirit. Through Contrology you first purposefully acquire complete control of your own body, and then through proper repetition of its exercises, you gradually and progressively acquire that natural rhythm and coordination associated with all your mental and subconscious activities." He went on to state that "Whole body health could be achieved through exercise, proper diet, good hygiene and sleeping habits, plenty of sunshine and fresh air, and a balance in life of work, recreation, and relaxation."[14]

I believe it is necessary for a movement practitioner to fully embrace the art and science of movement; it must integrate the mindful and spiritual roots we find in yoga, Pilates, martial arts, and other mindful movement forms. Each of the Principles of Movement you will read about in the following chapters is supported by scientific research and evidence-based outcomes. The intention was to create a series of movement principles that incorporate the science found in Western medicine, the growing body of energy medicine research, and the age-old practices dating back to the Vedas (Hindu scriptures that are the oldest archives of health and well-being known to man).

CONCLUSION

Before we start with the Principles of Movement, it is necessary to understand the importance movement awareness plays in learning, teaching, and correcting movement. My movement foundation is deeply rooted in the aspect of conscientious movement forms including dance, yoga, Pilates, the Feldenkrais Method, Gyrotonic Expansion System, and athletics. To achieve natural and spontaneous movement requires much more than objective measures, such as range of motion, repetitions, and isolated muscle torque. Each principle is built on the combination of quantitative measures and qualitative assessments. The combination of these 2 lenses when assessing, teaching, and facilitating change in movement can make all the difference. It is important to understand where movement awareness comes from historically and just how deep it runs in a human's right to move.

OPEN-ENDED QUESTIONS

1 Give an example of the difference between anatomy and functional anatomy. How can you apply functional anatomy to your own understanding of movement?

2 Reflect on a time where a lack of anatomical knowledge has impaired the quality of your own movement. What did you experience because of the lack of your own anatomical awareness?

3 How does congruency of joints improve energy efficiency?

4 Define the difference between osteokinematics and arthrokinematics.

5 Explain how understanding the arthrokinematics of a weight-bearing joint can influence quality of movement.

6 What is the difference between internal and external feedback? Which one represents more profound learning and is more likely to become spontaneous?

7 Describe the difference between motor control and motor learning. Which of these 2 sciences are we more likely to use as a movement facilitator? Why?

8 Describe in your own words how belief influences movement.

9 Give an example of how our mind can influence physical movement.

10 How can we use the mind and emotion to influence quality of movement?

11 Why is it important to understand this relationship between energies and energy fields as a movement practitioner?

12 List examples of ancient movement forms that embody bioenergetics and how you might draw on these older movement forms that can make you a better movement facilitator.

13 How does increased awareness of one's ability to move and where that movement comes from enhance the quality of movement?

REFERENCES

1. Franklin EN. *Conditioning for Dance*. Human Kinetics; 2004.

2. Comerford MJ, Mottram SL. Movement and stability dysfunction—contemporary developments. *Man Ther.* 2001;6(1):15-26.

3. Comerford MJ, Mottram SL. Functional stability re-training: principles and strategies for managing mechanical dysfunction. *Man Ther.* 2001;6(1):3-14.

4. Anderson BD. *Randomized Clinical Trial Comparing Active Versus Passive Approaches of the Treatment of Recurrent and Chronic Low Back Pain* [dissertation]. University of Miami; 2005.

5. Lackner JM, Carosella AM. The relative influence of perceived pain control, anxiety, and functional self efficacy on spinal function among patients with chronic low back pain. *Spine (Phila Pa 1976).* 1999;24(21):2254-2260; discussion 2260-2251.

6. Mannion AF, Junge A, Taimela S, Muntener M, Lorenzo K, Dvorak J. Active therapy for chronic low back pain: part 3. Factors influencing self-rated disability and its change following therapy. *Spine (Phila Pa 1976).* 2001;26(8):920-929.

7. Mannion AF, Taimela S, Muntener M, Dvorak J. Active therapy for chronic low back pain part 1. Effects on back muscle activation, fatigability, and strength. *Spine (Phila Pa 1976).* 2001;26(8):897-908.

8. Stolze LR, Allison SC, Childs JD. Derivation of a preliminary clinical prediction rule for identifying a subgroup of patients with low back pain likely to benefit from Pilates-based exercise. *J Orthop Sports Phys Ther.* 2012;42(5):425-436.

9. Bandura A. Health promotion by social cognitive means. *Health Educ Behav.* 2004;31(2):143-164.

10. Bandura A. Toward a psychology of human agency. *Perspect Psychol Sci.* 2006;1(2):164-180.

11. Bandura A. Toward a psychology of human agency: pathways and reflections. *Perspect Psychol Sci.* 2018;13(2):130-136.

12. Bandura A. Applying theory for human betterment. *Perspect Psychol Sci.* 2019;14(1):12-15.

13. Bandura A, Locke EA. Negative self-efficacy and goal effects revisited. *J Appl Psychol.* 2003;88(1):87-99.

14. Pilates JH, Miller WJ, Robbins J, Van Heuit-Robbins L. *Pilates Evolution: The 21st Century*. Presentation Dynamics; 2012.

15. National Center for Complementary and Integrative Health. https://www.nccih.nih.gov/health/complementary-alternative-or-integrative-health-whats-in-a-name

16. Borg-Olivier S. *Applied Anatomy & Physiology of Yoga*. Warisanoffset.com; 2006.

17. Alkadhi KA. Exercise as a positive modulator of brain function. *Mol Neurobiol.* 2018;55(4):3112-3130.

18. de Bruin EI, Formsma AR, Frijstein G, Bogels SM. Mindful2Work: effects of combined physical exercise, yoga, and mindfulness meditations for stress relieve in employees. A proof of concept study. *Mindfulness (N Y).* 2017;8(1):204-217.

QUALITATIVE VERSUS QUANTITATIVE MOVEMENT

QUALITATIVE MOVEMENT RELIES ON THE COMBINATION OF ACCURATE FEEDBACK, SELF-AWARENESS, AND PRACTICE SO THAT THE EXECUTION OF THE TASK IS SPONTANEOUS, EFFICIENT, AND REWARDING.

CHAPTER OBJECTIVES

1 Differentiate between qualitative movements and quantitative movements.

2 Acknowledge the connection between coaching self-awareness and increased efficiency of movement.

3 Appreciate the lessons learned from ancient and more modern movement forms that focus on qualitative movement (eg, yoga, Pilates, tai chi, Gyrotonic Expansion System, the Feldenkrais Method, ideokinesis).

KEY TERMS

- Apnea
- Awareness
- Bandhas
- External feedback
- Feldenkrais Method
- Gyrotonic Expansion System
- Ideokinesis
- Laban movement analysis
- Pranayama
- Qualitative movement
- Quantitative movement

Yoga, Pilates, the Feldenkrais Method, tai chi, ideokinesis, Laban movement analysis, and dance all can be considered conscientious movement forms that focus on elements of qualitative movement. This text introduces the difference between "qualitative" movement and "quantitative" movement, and more importantly, how they can be used together to improve the quality of our clients' and patients' lives. What differentiates a novice from an elite mover in all these movement forms? The answer is not necessarily found in the typical quantitative measures of outcome, such as range of motion or power to execute the desired movement. The difference can be determined by observing the quality of their movement. Qualitative movement is linked to the mover's ability to reflect on internal and external feedback mechanisms that improve performance. Movement performance relates to a particular task, with the intent of optimizing the movement efficiency within a defined

space. As a mover practices with well-guided internal and external feedback, they inherently improve the quality and effectiveness of their movement. The purpose of this text is to help us as movement practitioners tap into our client's self-awareness through coaching and meaningful feedback using the Principles of Movement to improve their quality of life. Lastly, this chapter focuses on the connection of body, mind, and spirit; we use the term *spirit* as it pertains to awareness.

As we entertain a deeper understanding of the factors that influence movement, we go back to some ancient movement forms found in yoga, martial arts (eg, kung fu, qigong, and tai chi), Oriental medicine, and Ayurvedic practices. This text also includes more recent qualitative movement forms, such as the Feldenkrais Method, Pilates, Laban movement analysis, Gyrotonic Expansion System, and ideokinesis, as well as forms of dance and

Anderson BD.
Principles of Movement (pp 14–22).
© 2024 Taylor & Francis Group.

sport that require higher-level body awareness and control. I have chosen yoga, Pilates, and the Feldenkrais Method to help establish the importance of mindfulness, awareness, and the quality of movement in this chapter.

YOGA

Yoga has been described as a practical approach to Ayurveda that can benefit psychophysical health.[1] The word yoga means union or to link together as one whole, incorporating body, mind, and spirit.[1-4] To separate the application of breath and the practice of movement and mindfulness would be a great disservice to the ancient art of yoga.

Yoga is the foundation of many movement forms practiced today, including martial arts, Pilates, Gyrotonic Expansion System, and various forms of dance. It has gained additional attention for its beneficial applications of breath, bandhas, posture, and ease of movement. Hatha yoga is one of the more popular yoga forms because it pertains to movement and the awareness of body, mind, and spirit. The original focus of hatha yoga was built on sedentary posture and poses, particularly the ability to sit for long periods of time.[1] It has been expanded to include postures of standing, supine, and prone and smooth transition through all the poses.

One of the key elements of yoga is breath. Breath is one of life's most essential needs, which goes without saying. The mastery seen in the practice of yoga breathing exercises (also known as *pranayama*) is much more than inhalation and exhalation.[1] The direction and timing of the breath, including the suspension of breath (apnea), have very meaningful purposes in the organization of body and mind control. In yoga, breath is referred to as *prana* or life's energy. It seems to me that the various applications of breath should be essential to all movement education methods. We dedicate an entire principle to breath and how breath facilitates movement and movement facilitates breath.

Other Principles of Movement that have a foundation in the practice of yoga are alignment, mobility, control, load, and coordination. Mindfulness of postural alignment before loading the tissues creates a natural and spontaneous organization of the neuromuscular system. Simon Borg-Olivier's definition of bandhas is a perfect way to understand how the contractile tissues (myofascial) create a cocontraction around joint complexes.[2] The anticipated load of a movement task, learned through previous experiences, will generate a cocontraction that provides stiffness around a joint complex.[2] This subconscious stiffness aids in maintaining congruence in the joints and the efficiency of the load placed on the elastic tissues.

Lastly, I want to address the mindfulness that is practiced in yoga and other meditative practices. In yoga, the meditative practice is referred to as *raja yoga* or the union of body and spirit by mental mastery.[1,2,5] Mindfulness, used in the context of awareness, is a powerful tool for teaching novel or corrective movement. According to the 4 stages of competence, there are stages of conscientious learning that can lead to unconscious and spontaneous performance.[6] Through the practice of movements in any sport or art form, one becomes increasingly efficient with the skills acquired. They progress from a state of unconscious incompetence to the highest level of performance of unconscious competence in which body and mind are efficiently one and are able to focus on a task with external feedback. Chapter 7 explains this motor learning model in greater depth.

THE PILATES METHOD

Joseph Pilates (Figure 2-1) was born in Germany in the late 1800s. He is the founder of Contrology, or Pilates as it is known today. Today, most Pilates teachers focus on the exercise repertoire of the Pilates method, but Joseph Pilates' philosophy was much more than just exercise. He was exposed to several movement forms, including yoga, calisthenics, and boxing. In Joseph Pilates' limited writings, he did emphatically express 3 guiding principles that required mindfulness and movement.[7]

In his first guiding principle, he wrote about whole body health and explained that it refers to the development of the body, the mind, and the spirit in complete coordination with each other. He wrote that whole body health could be achieved through exercise, proper diet, good hygiene and sleeping habits, plenty of sunshine and fresh air, and a balance in life of work, recreation, and relaxation.[7] The more I teach movement to restore health or rehabilitate impairments, the more I realize how important whole body health is. Movement cannot be about exercise alone and especially should not be isolated only into quantifiable movement factors, such as repetitions, ranges of motion, and quantities of load. Joseph Pilates further stated that "physical fitness is the first requisite of happiness. Our interpretation of physical fitness is the attainment and maintenance of a uniformly developed body with a sound mind, fully capable of naturally, easily, and satisfactorily performing our many and varied daily tasks with spontaneous zest and pleasure."[7] This is a powerful statement when applied to performance instruction or rehabilitation of movement-related pathologies. I am most impressed with his statement regarding "the ability to perform our many varied daily tasks naturally and spontaneously."[8] We have been overwhelmed with isolated core muscle training in our rehabilitation and fitness repertoire, which I believe often hampers the movement process. If we are doing our jobs as pathokinesiologists and performance kinesiologists correctly, we are facilitating our clients toward an unconscious performance of their many daily tasks with efficiency and the ability to be spontaneous in their adaptability. This is discussed in greater depth in the movement principle chapters.

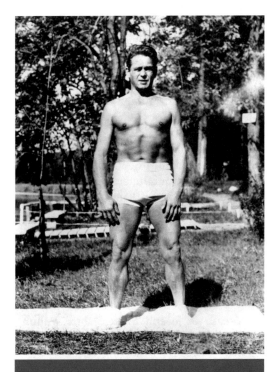

Figure 2-1. Joseph Pilates circa 1941.

Whole body commitment is Joseph Pilates' second guiding principle, which he defined as follows:

To achieve the highest accomplishments within the scope of our capabilities in all walks of life, we must constantly strive to acquire strong, healthy bodies and develop our minds to the limit of our ability. Whole body commitment is mental and physical discipline, a work ethic, and attitude toward oneself and assuming a lifestyle that is necessary to achieve whole body health.[7]

No matter what we believe is the right thing for our clients, if they do not learn to take responsibility and discipline themselves, they will not achieve the higher goals in their life, including happiness, according to Joseph Pilates.[9] In the International Classification of Functioning, Disability and Health by the World Health Organization, it becomes obvious that one of the key factors of influencing health is the patient's "participation."[10] This is what a patient chooses to participate in or believes they should be able to participate in. In our current health care system, the belief that our health insurance or government is solely responsible for our health or restoration of performance is a false expectation. Much of the responsibility lies in the individual and only the individual. Joseph Pilates' principle of whole body commitment resonates deeply with me as a physical therapist, and I realize that my job is to educate my patients so they can take responsibility for their personal well-being and hopefully control the expenses of maintaining healthy minds and bodies rather than the expensive costs of tertiary disease management.

Breath is Joseph Pilates' third guiding principle. Breath is an integral part of overall body function, managing tissue oxygenation, the removal of waste products, and even pH homeostasis. Full, consistent inhalation and exhalation help the circulatory system nourish all the tissues with oxygen-rich blood while carrying away impurities and metabolic waste. Joseph Pilates referred to this cleansing mechanism as the *internal shower*, which resulted in mental and physical invigoration and rejuvenation.[7] These teachings are deeply rooted in his hatha yoga training and are an essential part of every Pilates exercise. He had a few unique beliefs about breath. He believed that a full and complete exhalation would be able to clear out the germs that cause disease and move the air to prevent stagnation of disease. Much of his writing was done before the knowledge of microorganisms and antibiotics was commonplace. Current research shows the importance of breathing exercises as part of rehabilitation during and after respiratory disease or recovery from surgery. Although his highest priority is summed up in the quote "Above all, learn how to breathe correctly," there are very few specific instructions on breathing in his original work, unlike pranayama or qigong.

Joseph Pilates designed a system that is unique from the other movement methodologies; Pilates consists of equipment designed to provide a full spectrum of load and assistance in all orientations to gravity. This versatile property of Pilates is not commonly discussed but is a differentiator of his work. The unique design of Pilates equipment with springs and levers provides the practitioner with the ability to match the load exactly to what the client needs and progress the load to successfully acquire natural and spontaneous movement. Another area that is often overlooked was Joseph Pilates' desire for people to acquire the ability to participate in advanced human movement tasks (eg, squatting, jumping, crawling, climbing, wrestling, swinging, pulling, pushing). Many movement teachers think of Pilates as only the exercises on the mat and the machines, but his work went beyond this and is evident in film recordings of him conducting outdoor classes. He also believed in his essential formula of health and happiness, consisting of exercise, nutrition, sleep, hygiene, fresh air, sunshine, and a balance of life stressors (ie, work, play, and rest).[8] Many of the strategies and philosophies created by Joseph Pilates are used in this book to help the movement practitioner look at movement through a different lens.

There are many great leaders in qualitative movement from the early 20th century, including Mabel Elsworth Todd, Andre Bernard, Rudolf von Laban, Irmgard Bartenieff, Frederick Matthias Alexander, Martha Graham, Verne Inman, and so on. These pioneers focused on understanding movement acquisition, the quality of posture, movement, and the relationship between the body and the mind. One of my favorite pioneers of the 20th century is Moshe Feldenkrais. His focus on allowing movement exploration and discovery by the individual has greatly influenced my teaching.

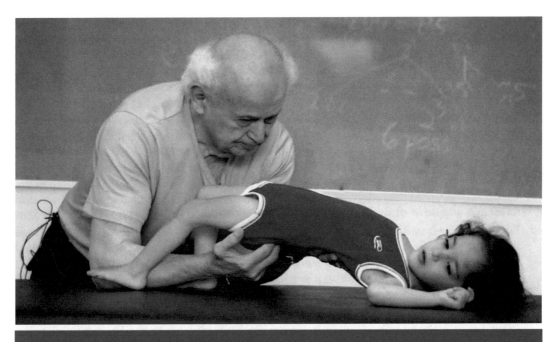

Figure 2-2. Moshe Feldenkrais. (© International Feldenkrais Federation.)

THE FELDENKRAIS METHOD

Dr. Moshe Feldenkrais (1904-1984; Figure 2-2), the founder of the Feldenkrais Method, was a physicist and judo master who applied his scientific mind to heal his own impairments from knee injuries and to help people reach their full potential.[11] Although it is difficult to identify specific guiding principles, as was done with the Pilates method, there are some fundamental ideas that Moshe Feldenkrais used in the development of the method. In this section, some of these foundational ideas are identified.

The Feldenkrais Method is an educational system that uses the fact that the body is the primary vehicle for learning. One often-quoted saying from Moshe Feldenkrais is "What I'm after isn't flexible bodies but flexible brains." Because he could not touch the person's brain directly, Moshe Feldenkrais developed this "brain flexibility" through differentiated, nonhabitual movements of the body. He developed 800+ lessons that set up a learning environment in which the person could learn to move in new nonhabitual patterns. The learning environments are structured to facilitate self-discovery and exploration, thereby improving the efficiency and clarity of how the person acts in the environment. Moshe Feldenkrais might not have used the term *neuroplasticity*, but he was one of the pioneers in using movements to influence changes in the nervous system. The Feldenkrais Method is not about removing movement patterns in the client but rather about giving people options on how to move, thereby expanding their movement repertoire, which will allow them to express themselves more fully and in a wider variety of contexts.[12]

The Feldenkrais Method is offered as lessons as opposed to treatments or exercises. Lessons are offered in the following 2 forms:

1. Awareness Through Movement encompasses verbally directed movement lessons in which subtleties of underlying movement patterns are explored to create profound shifts in the overall efficiency of movement. The lessons are usually taught in a group environment. The results include greater comfort, ease, performance, and sense of well-being.[13]

2. Functional Integration is a one-on-one hands-on approach in which the practitioner uses their hands to provide feedback to inform the student and explore efficient paths of movement. Unlike massage, the person is clothed, and the practitioner is focusing on movement patterns throughout the body as a whole.

Another foundational idea of the Feldenkrais Method is that movements will be performed slowly and with minimal effort. As a scientist, Moshe Feldenkrais was aware of the Weber-Fechner law, and he applied that law to human movement. The law basically states that the stronger the stimulus is, the less sensitive we are to small differences, and the weaker the stimulus, the more sensitive we are to small differences. It is easy to sense the difference of an increase of 1 kg if the weight we are lifting is 2 kg, but if the weight we are lifting is 100 kg, then it is more difficult to feel the addition of 1 kg. The more effort we use in our movements, the less we can detect small differences. To take that concept one step further, the more force we use, the more likely we are to use habitual movements; therefore, no learning of new movements takes place. We go to the default movement when more force is needed. For the nervous system to learn something new, initially the movement should be performed slowly and with minimal effort.[14]

To be able to change habits in movement as well as thinking and breathing patterns, the student must first be able to recognize the habitual pattern. One of the more famous quotes from Moshe Feldenkrais is the following: "If you don't know what you are doing, you can't do what you want." How can we change the way we move unless we are aware of the habitual way that we are moving? One of the first things that happens in a Feldenkrais Method lesson is to have the student recognize/identify their habitual pattern. The student is then guided through alternative ways to move. They learn to notice the difference between the habitual movement pattern and alternative pattern when performing an action/function, such as sitting, crawling, walking, or reaching. This is important because we need to be able to perform a specific action in a variety of ways depending on the situation/context we are in. Moshe Feldenkrais realized how our habitual patterns influence our emotional state and that each emotional state has a specific pattern of muscular contraction. By developing different ways of moving, we develop different patterns of muscular contractions, thereby allowing us to develop/reach more emotional states. Moving, sensing, thinking, and feeling are inseparable in reality, so Feldenkrais Method students and clients often report that improvements in habits, movement, and perception lead them to feel more flexible, responsive, and expressive in their thinking and emotional lives.[13] The Feldenkrais Method views the whole as a unity and does not separate the person into physical, emotional, and spiritual aspects.

Previously in this chapter, I quoted Moshe Feldenkrais stating that he was not after flexible bodies but flexible brains. However, we must not forget the last part of that quote—"What I'm after is to restore each person to their human dignity." This is what he was really after, and I think it connects him with Joseph Pilates in that he stated "the ability to perform our many varied daily tasks naturally and spontaneously."[8] If we perform our many varied daily tasks naturally and spontaneously, we perform them with dignity.

OPEN-ENDED QUESTIONS

1 Differentiate between qualitative and quantitative movement.

2 How can we measure qualitative movements?

3 Explain the effects of a bandha in physiological terms.

4 How might mindfulness of a novel movement or corrective movement facilitate a more natural motor pattern?

5 Joseph Pilates' philosophy focused on the ability for one to perform their many varied daily tasks naturally and spontaneously. How might you apply this to your life, sports, and rehabilitation? How might this apply to working with clients or patients?

6 What are some unique designs within Joseph Pilates' equipment and method that facilitate early mindful learning of movement, particularly with novice movement or restoration of movement following pathology? How would you explain this to a friend or colleague?

7 Explain how the Feldenkrais Method of "awareness through movement" might differ from more traditional athletic training and rehabilitation techniques.

8 Describe in your own words how you as a pathokinesiologist or performance kinesiologist can incorporate feeling, awareness, and internal feedback into your practice.

REFERENCES

1. Hewitt J. *The Complete Yoga Book: Yoga of Breathing, Yoga of Posture, and Yoga of Meditation*. Schocken Books; 1978.

2. Borg-Olivier S. *Applied Anatomy & Physiology of Yoga*. Warisanoffset.com; 2006.

3. Feuerstein G. *The Philosophy of Classical Yoga*. Inner Traditions International; 1996.

4. Feuerstein G. *The Shambhala Guide to Yoga*. 1st ed. Shambhala; 1996.

5. Yogananda. *Autobiography of a Yogi*. Crystal Clarity Publishers; 1946.

6. Flower J. In the mush. *Physician Exec*. 1999;25(1):64-66.

7. Pilates JH, Miller WJ, Robbins J, Van Heuit-Robbins L. *Pilates Evolution: The 21st Century*. Presentation Dynamics; 2012.

8. Lederman E. The fall of the postural-structural-biomechanical model in manual and physical therapies: exemplified by lower back pain. *J Bodyw Mov Ther*. 2011;15(2):131-138.

9. Pilates JH. *Return to Life Through Contrology*. J. J. Augustin Publisher; 1945.

10. Heinemann AW, Magasi S, Bode RK, et al. Measuring enfranchisement: importance of and control over participation by people with disabilities. *Arch Phys Med Rehabil*. 2013;94(11):2157-2165.

11. Reese M. *Moshe Feldenkrais: A Life in Movement*. ReeseKress Somatics Press; 2015.

12. AmericaFeldenkrais Guild of North America. Standard of practice. 2022. Accessed April 18, 2022. https://cdn.ymaws.com/feldenkrais.site-ym.com/resource/resmgr/pdf/02-28-22-standards-of-practi.pdf

13. Feldendrais MB. *Embodied Wisdom: The Collected Papers of Moshe Feldenkrais*. North Atlantic Books; 2010.

14. Smyth C. Practical maturity. In: Elgelid S, Kresge C, eds. *The Feldenkrais Method: Learning Through Movement*. Handspring Press; 2021.

BREATH

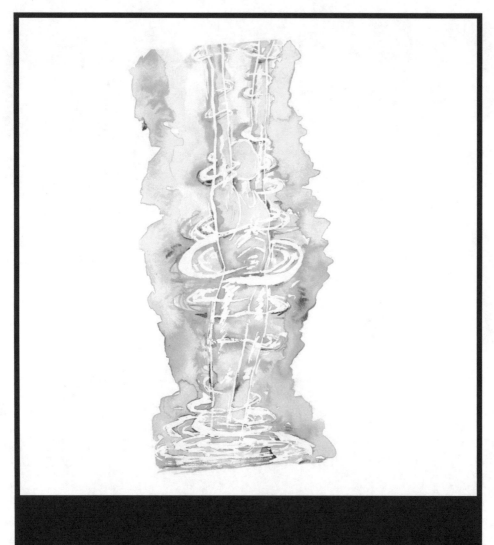

**BREATH FACILITATES MOVEMENT AND
MOVEMENT FACILITATES BREATH.**

CHAPTER OBJECTIVES

1 Recognize the effectiveness of breath in movement assessment and facilitation.

2 Describe the 3-dimensional thorax movement that breath can facilitate.

3 Assess a client's breathing bias and what ramifications that bias may have on the client's movement.

4 Facilitate breath in all 3 dimensions of the lungs and chest.

5 Demonstrate how breath can facilitate movement and how movement can facilitate breath.

6 Explain the effect of the neuromusculoskeletal system on breathing and how breathing directly influences the neuromusculoskeletal system.

7 Explain the physiology of breathing as it pertains to gas exchange.

KEY TERMS

- Accessory breathing
- Aponeurosis
- Axial elongation
- Carbon dioxide (CO_2)
- Costovertebral joint
- Crura of the diaphragm
- Diaphragm
- Expiration
- Flared rib cage
- Hydraulic amplifier
- Hyperventilation
- Inspiration
- Intra-abdominal pressure
- Pleura
- Prana
- Pranayama
- Respiration
- Rule of the ribs
- Thorax
- Tidal volume

One of the most important principles of facilitating movement is breath. Breath is the essence of life and life's energy. It has been used in many ancient and modern movement and healing art forms. Through a deeper understanding of breath and the anatomy, physiology, and biomechanics of the thorax, it becomes evident that a simple understanding of breath can be a powerful tool in facilitating movement.

BREATH FACILITATES MOVEMENT AND MOVEMENT FACILITATES BREATH.

Breath, the age-old principle present in every movement methodology, can be thought of as one of the great facilitators of movement. Scientifically, we refer to it as *respiration*. In spiritual writings, breath is frequently related to life (eg, "the breath of life," "living breath," and "God breathed life into man."[1]).

Anderson BD.
Principles of Movement (pp 24-54).
© 2024 Taylor & Francis Group.

Sally was a patient of mine who suffered from a serious autonomic nerve syndrome known as *complex regional pain syndrome* (CRPS) after a severe motor vehicle accident. This syndrome caused severe pain and hypersensitivity to any touch of her right hand. As a result, she stopped using her right arm and shoulder and subconsciously changed her breathing pattern into what was probably a protective pattern. She began to use her anterior cervical muscles to "lift" her ribs to assist in breathing instead of allowing her lower ribs to expand. This complicated her symptoms. Breathing in this accessory pattern was very inefficient and resulted in fatigue, slower healing, and emotional frustration. Another side effect of using these accessory muscles to breathe is the pressure they place on the nerves and vascular structures that correspond to the arm from the brachial plexus.

I saw Sally after she failed many different interventions, including nerve block injections, implanted drug feeding devices, desensitization programs, and psychological counseling for pain management. I realized that all the traditional approaches for treating CRPS that I had learned were not helping Sally; yet, I believed that an answer existed. As I listened to her, I was able to uncover other psychosocial factors that influenced her dysfunctions. CRPS can be defined as a faulty loop or wiring of the sympathetic nervous system. The sympathetic nervous system is often associated with fight, fright, and flight behavior. The simple act of going on the web or reading a book on CRPS can increase the fear around this diagnosis and exacerbate symptoms. Sally's partner did not understand the nature of the impairment, and because he could not see it, he discredited her complaints as psychological. Sally's repeated treatment failures increased her fear and discouragement.

I felt strongly that what Sally really needed was to have a successful movement experience, and yet, according to Sally, all movement reproduced pain; therefore, she was apprehensive. I concluded that the first step would be to provide a successful breathing experience and

move forward from there. I used a relaxation technique I had learned years before, shifting attention from the affected limb to gentle movement of the ribs through the exchange of air. After 5 or 6 sessions, she noticed a tapering of the pain, and I noticed new movement in the thorax when she was in this relaxed state. I started combining the relaxation techniques with directional breathing and noticed that her breath was facilitating movement in her entire body. Inhalation facilitated extension of the thoracic spine and an upward rotation of the ribs, which led to a gentle extension of the lower back, an anterior tilt of the pelvis, and an internal rotation of the femurs. Exhalation facilitated the opposite movement of the spine and pelvis into flexion. Breathing into one lung facilitated side bending of the spine, and breathing into her right lung was beneficial for Sally because getting movement around her sympathetic ganglia without pain or an increase in pain was a big step for her. Although I originally had no intention of putting Sally on the Pilates equipment, I now saw an opportunity. If I could facilitate the same patterns of movement on the Pilates equipment, I could potentially create an environment for her to find a movement pattern that did not increase her pain and could improve her strategies. Over the next 3 months, Sally was able to gradually perform more of her daily activities with confidence and started to believe that not all movement was associated with pain. When she did have pain, she had a new strategy to control it with relaxation, breathing, and gentle movement of her body. The focus of her treatment progressed to alignment, efficiency of movement, and self-awareness.

Years later, I was teaching anatomy at the University of Miami and assisting with a lab in which we dissected a thorax. As we sectioned the thorax and moved past the heart, lung, and circulatory systems, we came to the sympathetic ganglia (Figure 3-1), which happens to rest on top of the joints connecting the ribs to the vertebrae that create the 12 costovertebral junctions. I had a flashback to Sally. It was one of those moments when you hit your forehead and say to yourself "of course!" Whether Sally had a postural dysfunction before the spine injury from the motor vehicle accident that resulted in CRPS or a faulty breathing pattern that preceded the motor vehicle accident, I will never know, but I do feel that the attention to breath, posture, and gentle successful movement was the solution to Sally's dysfunction.[2] I have since had numerous experiences with my patients in which breath facilitation was an essential factor in restoring healthy movement, especially for those who had given up hope of getting better.

Breath is a facilitator for stabilization and mobilization of the spine. Pilates, yoga, Gyrotonic Expansion System, and qigong movements create an environment in which breathing is used to increase breath capacity, increase the efficiency of gas exchange, and facilitate thoracic postural changes. We find that many clients suffering from common spinal injuries have a decrease in thoracic spine and rib mobility. Faulty breath patterns have been clinically associated with common complaints of pain and movement dysfunction. Although the approach to breathing varies depending on the methodology, they share a common thread—breath is an integral part of movement. *Breath facilitates movement and movement facilitates breath.*

Breath can only occur in 2 ways: through movement of the diaphragm or movement of the rib cage. We do not breathe through our skin, eyes, or other parts of our body. Breath only occurs through the displacement of the rib cage and the diaphragm. Interestingly, around the world, in many cultures and movement forms, breath has many more applications besides just exchanging gases.[3]

In pranayama practice, breath is used to change energy levels, improve digestion, facilitate movement, and connect spiritually to the source. According to Simon Borg-Olivier, yoga is the art of learning how to regulate and be comfortable with one's breath in all situations. The purpose of deep breathing is not to take in more air but rather to aerate those parts of the lungs that are not aerated in everyday

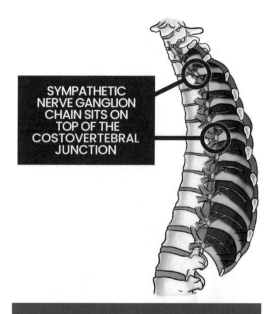

SYMPATHETIC NERVE GANGLION CHAIN SITS ON TOP OF THE COSTOVERTEBRAL JUNCTION

Figure 3-1. Sympathetic ganglia.

breathing. Breathing is the art of learning how to make the most effective use of every bit of both the air that we breathe in and the prana we absorb.[4] I love this interpretation of breath because it has many purposes and can be thought of as a tool not a rule.

Blandine Calais-Germain stated in her 2006 book, *Anatomy of Breathing*, that there are many applications of breath outside of exchanging air, including vocalization, energy shifts, pleasure, pain management, facilitation of movement, exercise of rib cage control, and accentuation or moderation of the curvature of the spine.[3] She goes on further to state that complex movements require spontaneous breath.

In his 1945 book, *Return to Life Through Contrology*, Joseph Pilates said the following: "… your blood will flow with renewed vigor as a direct result of your faithfully performing the Contrology exercises. These exercises induce the heart to pump strong and steadily. As a result, the bloodstream carries and discharges from your system more of the accumulated debris created by fatigue."[5,6]

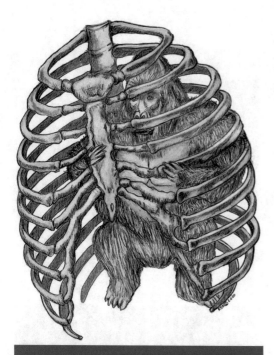

Figure 3-2. A gorilla in the rib cage.
(Illustrated by Kelly Anderson.)

Joseph Pilates knew that the movement of breath and stimulation of the circulatory system were essential for health. It becomes evident that breath in its physiological, mechanical, energetic, and spiritual applications is and should be the center of our movement principles. For these reasons, breath earns the first position in the Polestar Principles of Movement.

ESSENTIAL SCIENCES
FUNCTIONAL ANATOMY OF BREATHING

We begin to explore the complexities and beauty of breath by looking at the anatomy. Starting with the skeletal structures of breath, the thoracic cage (also known as the *rib cage*) is probably the most important. When I typically think of a cage, I imagine an enclosure at the

zoo with an 800-pound gorilla on the other side (Figure 3-2). I do not want the bars of that cage or enclosure to move or be flexible. However, when we speak of the rib cage, we can think of a spring-loaded structure that has 12 articulating vertebrae that move in all planes with 12 flexible ribs attached on either side. The ribs contain the highest percentage of elastin and are the most flexible bones in the body. The ribs are connected to a floating bone called the *sternum* through rubbery cartilage. The rib cage protects the vital organs, including the heart, lungs, and liver, in the thorax and is a stable structure that is a perfect balance between stiffness and flexibility (Figures 3-3A and 3-3B).

When the thorax is mobile, it can be part of an efficient, synergistic system that distributes forces to and from the surrounding tissues. If movement is not happening in the thoracic spine and rib cage, it must happen elsewhere, which is often the shoulders, neck, or lumbar spine (structures that are not meant to move without a supple thorax). Limited breath capacity in the different planes of movement can often be associated with an increased risk of pathology and disease.

The next important structure is the diaphragm. The diaphragm enlarges the volume of the thoracic cavity, forcing the lungs to expand (Figures 3-4A and 3-4B). Anteriorly, it attaches to the inferior border of the rib cage just behind the sternum at the level of the 7th rib and connects to the lowest ribs all the way around toward the spine at the level of the 12th thoracic vertebra. The domes of the diaphragm rest approximately at T4 and when contracted can descend approximately 7 cm.[7] The aponeurosis, the connective covering of the diaphragm, is connected to the pleura, which surrounds the lungs. When the diaphragm contracts, it lowers and pulls on the pleura, which changes the shape of the lungs, decreases the internal pressure, and facilitates inhalation. A common misconception is that as we inhale, the diaphragm is pushed down with the air we are moving into the lungs. Instead, the contraction of the diaphragm is what initiates the movement of air into the lungs.

[A]
ANTERIOR RIB CAGE

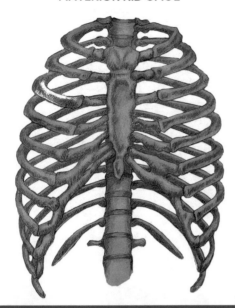

[B]
POSTERIOR RIB CAGE

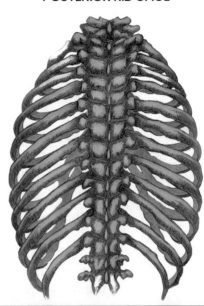

Figure 3-3. The (A) anterior rib cage and (B) posterior rib cage. (Illustrated by Kelly Anderson.)

During the concentric contraction, the diaphragm moves inferiorly and anteriorly. The organs that lie directly underneath the diaphragm are displaced with every contraction and every breath. There is no empty space between the diaphragm and the viscera below. Therefore, we see outward movement of the abdominal wall when the diaphragm contracts to inhale. When the diaphragm relaxes, it returns to its dome-like position, increasing the pressure in the lungs and facilitating exhalation. The diaphragm works automatically and subconsciously. Resting breath, which is also known as *tidal volume*, is the amount of air exchanged during a resting unconscious breath (eg, while we sleep or as you read this book).

Notice the crura of the diaphragm in Figure 3-4C. These are musculotendinous slips that are called *arcuate ligaments*; they create openings or apertures. These apertures are the openings that permit the large vessels to pass from the upper thoracic cavity to the abdominal cavity.[8] These vessels include the vena cava, descending aorta, and esophagus.

Each crus connects to the lumbar vertebrae and the anterior longitudinal ligament approximately at the levels of L4-5. This is a very important factor in understanding the role of breath and the diaphragm in relation to trunk stability and control. The apex of the lumbar lordotic curve is around L3. The crura of the diaphragm connect to the anterior part of the lumbar spine just below the apex. This understanding of the anatomy makes it easier to understand how the contraction of the diaphragm combined with subconscious contractions of the abdominal wall, especially the transverse abdominis, facilitate the axial length of the spine and can aid in decreasing lumbar lordosis. If the diaphragm works by itself without the force couples of the transverse abdominis, lumbar multifidus, and pelvic floor in a vertically loaded posture,

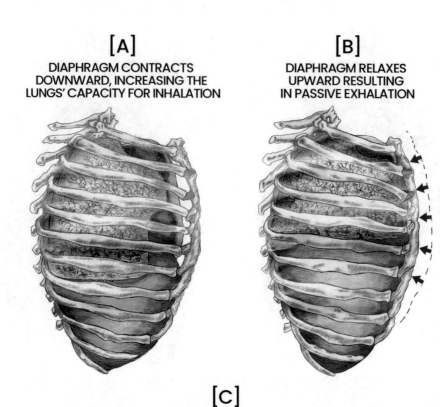

[A]
DIAPHRAGM CONTRACTS
DOWNWARD, INCREASING THE
LUNGS' CAPACITY FOR INHALATION

[B]
DIAPHRAGM RELAXES
UPWARD RESULTING
IN PASSIVE EXHALATION

[C]
INFERIOR DIAPHRAGM

CENTRAL TENDON

VENA CAVA

ESOPHAGUS

DESCENDING AORTA

PSOAS MAJOR MUSCLE

QUADRATUS LUMBORUM MUSCLE

CRURA OF THE DIAPHRAGM

Figure 3-4. (A) The diaphragm contracts downward, increasing the lungs' capacity for inhalation. (B) The diaphragm relaxes upward, resulting in passive exhalation. (C) The diaphragm.

(Illustrated by Kelly Anderson.)

it can actually result in exaggerated lumbar lordosis or an anterior shift of the thorax.[9] This increase in lordosis at end-range extension can lead to unwanted anterior shear force. Anterior shear force can happen when the vertebrae slide horizontally, potentially resulting in a compromise of the vertebral foramina. It is through these vertebral foramina that the nerve roots pass, and they contain sensory and motor tracts to and from the lower extremities (in this case, levels L3-4, L4-5, and L5-S1). This is why good organization of the torso and diaphragm is so crucial for healthy alignment of the spine.[10] The psoas major and quadratus lumborum muscles also pass through the ligamentous openings posterior to the diaphragm and attach to the transverse vertebral processes and the anterior costovertebral junctions above the T12 vertebra (see Figure 3-4C). There is a relationship between the most medial fibers of the hip flexors, quadratus lumborum, diaphragm, and the pelvic floor that dynamically provide stiffness to the trunk, particularly the connection between the pelvis and the thoracic spine. The pubococcygeus muscle's posterior fibers insert into the anterior longitudinal

ligament in the same fascial layer as the crura of the diaphragm. Three-dimensionally, the diaphragm, hip flexors, multifidus, pelvic floor, and anterior wall of the abdomen, including the oblique abdominals and the transverse abdominis, create a hydraulic amplifier. The hydraulic amplifier model, also known as the *intra-abdominal pressure (IAP) model* (Figure 3-5), serves to connect the thorax with the pelvis and to protect the lumbar spine by maintaining the appropriate amount of stiffness and IAP required by the anticipated movement task or activity. The important thing to understand is that the muscles of the hydraulic amplifier work subconsciously and at a submaximal contraction in response to the anticipated load of a desired task or activity.[11,12] This means that the amount of engagement will vary and automatically change based on what we are doing. What an amazing system!

A common misconception about core control exercises is that we are to contract the abdominal wall all the time (ie, the more the better). Feel the burn. This engaging and holding of the abdominal wall can interfere

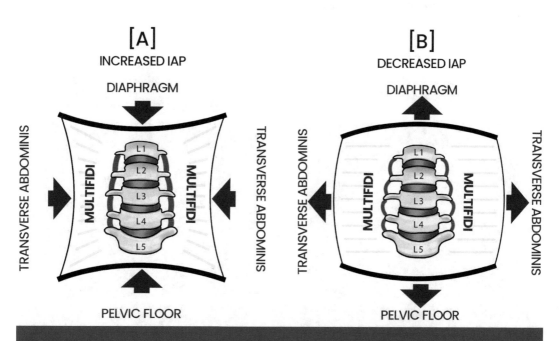

Figure 3-5. The hydraulic amplifier.

with efficient movement and impair digestion, respiration, and pelvic floor function. All muscles need to contract and relax to be healthy, including the abdominal wall. In many Western exercises, the emphasis is primarily on voluntary contractions, and we often hear "squeeze your abs" or "pull in your abs." When we study movement forms like tai chi, qigong, and forms of yoga, they teach us that we must be able to allow the abdominal wall to expand with deep breathing. This can be observed in many forms of meditation as well. In Pilates, the concept of the "powerhouse" that Joseph Pilates often referred to has been misinterpreted by some to mean always contracting the anterior abdominal wall and always funneling the rib cage. The 2 activities require an over-recruitment of the oblique abdominal muscles, particularly the internal obliques. I have seen clients who have strategized in this way for so long that they developed a contracture of the anterior abdominal wall and can no longer allow the abdominal muscles to lengthen enough to take in a deep breath. In 2015, we collected data on the ability of female Pilates teachers to voluntarily contract their pelvic floor muscles, particularly

the pubococcygeus muscle. Historically, many movement practitioners, therapists, nurses, and doctors have taught pelvic floor exercises by cueing volitional tightening or lifting of the pelvic floor muscles (Kegels). In our study, we wanted to know if Pilates teachers could accurately activate the pelvic floor muscles. If there were a group of individuals who should know how to activate their pelvic floor, it theoretically should be Pilates teachers. We recruited 45 experienced female Pilates teachers. Each was asked to voluntarily lift their pelvic floor muscles up. On observation with ultrasound, we saw 21 of them (almost half) either pushed their pelvic floor down or did not have a contraction at all (Figures 3-6A and 3-6B). Interestingly, when they were cued to take a full breath in and out, the movement of the pelvic floor muscles responded correctly in 95% of the teachers. With inhalation, the pelvic floor descended, and with exhalation, the pelvic floor ascended. Based on these outcomes, I would propose that volitional cueing of the pelvic floor often does not result in the desired outcome of spontaneously and correctly activating the pelvic floor. Think how many women suffer from incontinence when

[A]

NORMAL ELEVATION
WITH CONTRACTION

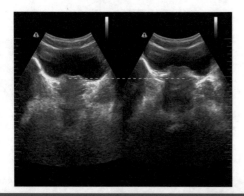

[B]

PELVIC FLOOR DESCENDED
WHEN SUBJECT THOUGHT THEY
WERE ELEVATING PELVIC FLOOR

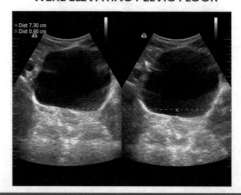

Figure 3-6. (A) An ultrasound of the pelvic floor showing normal elevation with contraction. (B) An ultrasound of the pelvic floor showing the pelvic floor descended when the participant thought they were elevating the pelvic floor.

engaging in an activity such as lifting a child. Would the outcome be different if they were simply aware of their breath during these movements? Movement of the diaphragm can influence movement of the pelvic floor; they work synergistically to regulate IAP. Research has shown that voluntary contractions of posture muscles can interfere with the natural and spontaneous neuromuscular organization of the thorax and pelvic musculature.[13] Are we accidentally cueing our clients to make their movement less efficient?

When we look at the muscles that are responsible for moving the rib cage during breath (Figures 3-7A through 3-7D), they include the intercostal muscles, the abdominal muscles, the serratus posterior superior and inferior muscles, the levator costarum muscles, and the accessory breath muscles, including the scalene and sternocleidomastoid muscles. These muscles work synergistically to move the rib cage.

INSPIRATION

The diaphragm and the external intercostals are inspiratory muscles that when contracted cause the expansion of the thorax. The external intercostals help to lift and expand the ribs outward and upward, and the diaphragm moves downward. The serratus posterior superior and inferior aid in the force couple of both inhalation and exhalation. As mentioned previously, a pressure change is created when these muscles contract, which brings air into the lungs.

Another group of inspiratory muscles are the accessory breath muscles (see Figure 3-7D), which consist of the sternocleidomastoids, the scalenes, and the other anterior strap muscles of the neck. Although not typically thought of as being efficient breathing muscles, these muscles can change the shape of the superior rib cage and create enough pressure change to help exchange air. Accessory breathing is often associated with faulty breathing patterns,

especially if it is the primary strategy for resting breath. We often observe this pattern in smokers and individuals with very poor posture. We are also noting more accessory breathing with exercise enthusiasts who want the image of a narrow rib cage and skinny waist. The problem with this type of breathing is that it can often lead to secondary problems in the cervical spine. One of the most common problems with accessory breathing is the constriction it creates around the brachial plexus between the scalene muscles. This can lead to radiating pain down the arm and eventually serious pathologies, such as CRPS, which was discussed previously. One might ask why we were born with accessory breathing mechanisms if it is so inefficient and potentially harmful to us. The answer is in the name "accessory." Imagine being at the end of a marathon, and you need just a little more oxygen (O_2) to make it through the finish line; this type of breathing can come in handy. In spinal cord injuries above C3, the only type of breathing available is accessory because the other muscles are paralyzed. Actor Christopher Reeve suffered a C2 fracture and only had accessory breathing capabilities; he required a respirator most of the time. When the respirator was removed, he could only sustain his air intake for a short period of time through accessory breathing. Individuals with asthma and chronic obstructive pulmonary disease (COPD)–type conditions use this strategy of breathing when they are unable to breathe with the normal expansion of the ribs and lungs. Accessory breathing has its place, but it does not achieve what Joseph Pilates referred to as the *internal shower*. Not being able to fully exhale and have good air exchange may lead to an increased incidence of respiratory infections because the lack of internal cleansing of pathogens and waste products can be trapped in parts of the lung that experience poor circulation, as found in COPD, and lead to disease and illness. One of the most common causes of death in the hospital is respiratory failure caused by pneumonia. I believe this is because of our inability to facilitate full and complete breaths, as Joseph Pilates described in his image of the internal shower.

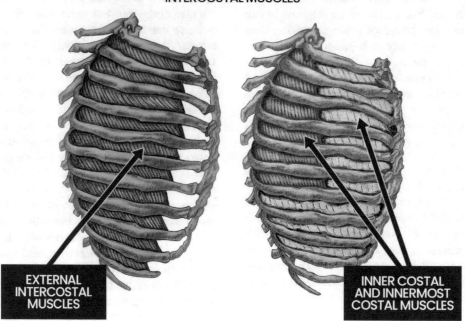

[A]
INTERCOSTAL MUSCLES

EXTERNAL INTERCOSTAL MUSCLES

INNER COSTAL AND INNERMOST COSTAL MUSCLES

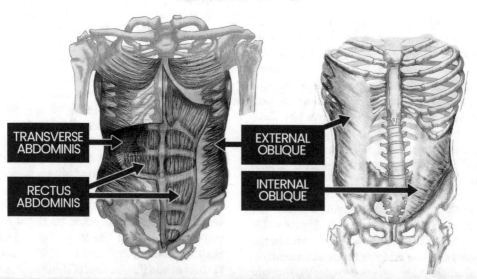

[B]
ABDOMINAL MUSCLES

TRANSVERSE ABDOMINIS

RECTUS ABDOMINIS

EXTERNAL OBLIQUE

INTERNAL OBLIQUE

Figure 3-7. The breathing muscles: (A) the intercostal muscles and (B) abdominal muscles. (continued)

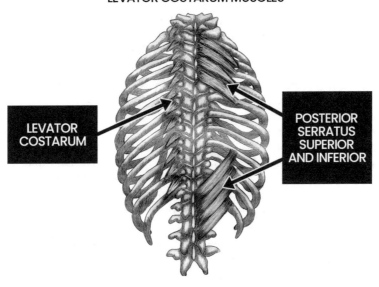

[C]
POSTERIOR SERRATUS AND
LEVATOR COSTARUM MUSCLES

LEVATOR COSTARUM

POSTERIOR SERRATUS SUPERIOR AND INFERIOR

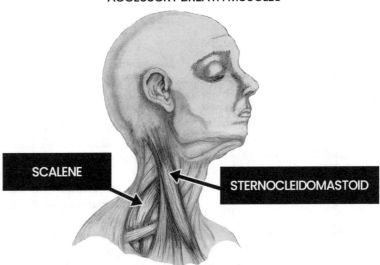

[D]
ACCESSORY BREATH MUSCLES

SCALENE

STERNOCLEIDOMASTOID

Figure 3-7 (continued). The breathing muscles: (C) posterior serratus and levator costarum muscles and (D) accessory breath muscles. (Illustrated by Kelly Anderson.)

EXPIRATION

Muscles of expiration consist primarily of the abdominal muscles, the internal intercostal muscles, and the serratus posterior muscles, which contribute to the force couple of rib movement (see Figure 3-7C). When the abdominal muscles contract, they narrow the abdomen and the base of the rib cage. This increases IAP, pushes the viscera up underneath the relaxing diaphragm, and increases the pressure inside the lungs, facilitating exhalation. The inner intercostal muscles, which run in the same plane as the internal abdominal obliques, are in the lower ribs. When the inner intercostal muscles contract, they draw the ribs down, increasing the narrowing pressure of the thorax and facilitating exhalation. The intercostal muscles can only work if there is an equal and opposite force superiorly, which allows the lower ribs to move inferiorly, toward the cage inferiorly, and toward the central axis. Pranayama practice in a sitting position demonstrates the importance of spine length to optimize the breath[14] because when the spine is axially elongated, the muscles and fascia organize themselves naturally to allow the rib cage to move efficiently and dynamically. Good posture during breathing can be one of the best ways to facilitate healthy and easy inhalation and exhalation. Slouch and try to take in a full breath, and then sit up and do the same thing. Good vertical posture provides greater capacity of movement in all planes during breath; the diaphragm can descend lower, and the ribs and the thoracic spine can have greater displacement, creating greater displacement of the lungs both in inhalation and exhalation.

On each end of the thorax and abdomen are 2 more diaphragms. Above the lungs and thorax are the vocal cords (Figure 3-8), and below the abdominal cavity is the pelvic floor (Figure 3-9). These areas can have a direct effect on breath, movement, and stability because of the pressure they exert on the lungs and abdomen.

The vocal cords are often used by Alexander Technique, Pilates, and Feldenkrais Method teachers as a way to sustain abdominal pressure through a movement sequence.[15] The contraction of the vocal cords and/or the pursing of one's lips can control the amount and duration of air that escapes, providing more control of the IAP. Kathy Grant studied with Joseph Pilates and taught at the New York University Tisch School of the Arts. She had her students sing and recite their address while performing certain Pilates exercises, such as the roll up. Singing and speaking ensure that the IAP stays constant and can significantly improve the quality of movement. You cannot hold your breath and force your way through the movement. Closing the epiglottis and holding the breath or even exhaling quickly and not having any air left in the lungs significantly reduces the quality of movement, especially movement that requires spine articulation.

To experience how breathing and holding the breath influence movement, take a moment and perform the roll up exercise (Figures 3-10A through 3-10C) using the singing breath pattern described in Box 3-1 to feel the consistency or lack of consistency of IAP.

As discussed earlier, the pelvic floor is an area of great interest in breath and core control. I often feel that we have overemphasized trying to voluntarily recruit the pelvic floor muscles to increase core control. As with many of the deep muscles of the trunk, these muscles have been shown to function subconsciously and submaximally.[16,17]

I am not belittling the importance of the pelvic floor muscles, as a matter of fact just the opposite. They play a very important role in breath, control, and posture. I use breath, alignment, and load as movement modalities to influence a normal spontaneous contraction of the pelvic floor and other postural muscles of the trunk. This is addressed further in Chapter 6, in which the principle of control is discussed. One of the pelvic floor's roles is to provide dynamic pressure from the bottom of the abdomen when IAP must be maintained

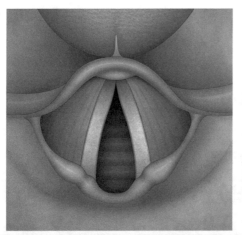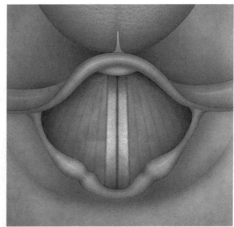

Figure 3-8. The vocal cords.

(Aldona Griskeviciene/Shutterstock.com.)

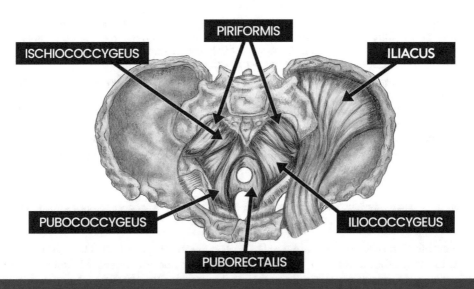

PIRIFORMIS

ISCHIOCOCCYGEUS

ILIACUS

PUBOCOCCYGEUS

ILIOCOCCYGEUS

PUBORECTALIS

Figure 3-9. The pelvic floor muscles.

(Illustrated by Kelly Anderson.)

over a sustained period. The Pilates exercise called *the hundred* is breath-centric and a perfect example of this (Figure 3-11).

The goal or purpose of the hundred is to maintain the body position and breathe in and out 20 times while beating the arms 100 times (a grouping of 5 arm beats to 1 inhalation and 5 beats to 1 exhalation), hence the name the hundred. It seems easy enough, but there are

many factors increasing the challenge. The legs extended parallel to the floor provide a constant load on the trunk and hip flexor muscles. The curl up or chest lift position requires the use of the abdominal muscles, and then there is the coordination of the breath and the pumping of the arms. Teachers often wrongly cue a strong contraction of the abdominal muscles that makes air exchange almost impossible. Remember the diaphragm

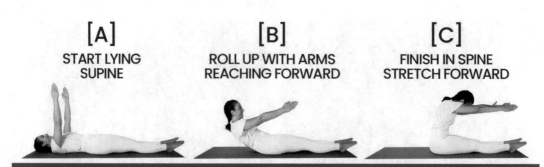

[A]
START LYING
SUPINE

[B]
ROLL UP WITH ARMS
REACHING FORWARD

[C]
FINISH IN SPINE
STRETCH FORWARD

Figure 3-10. A Pilates roll up. (A) Start lying in supine. (B) Roll up with the arms reaching forward. (C) Finish in the long sit position.

BOX 3-1: THE ROLL UP

Singing or talking out loud provides a steady flow of air and can optimize spine mobility and fluidity in the roll up exercise. Conversely, performing the roll up exercise while performing a Valsalva (ie, strongly holding the breath) greatly restricts spine mobility. In this experience, perform the roll up with both techniques.

1. Hold your breath while rolling up, breathe in again at the top, and hold your breath on the roll down.

2. Sing from 1 to 8 while rolling up and from 8 to 1 while rolling down (eg, do-re-mi). Ensure that the voice quality is the same with every number that is sung and that the count covers the entire movement in tempo. Sing loud and strong.

Observation: Did you observe a difference in mobility, ease, and power? If so, which one was easier for you?

needs to be able to move. To maintain a safe IAP when inhaling, the abdominal wall and pelvic floor muscles must eccentrically contract or lengthen to maintain dynamic constant pressure to sustain a constant load. When the exhalation occurs, the opposite happens; the diaphragm relaxes, and the abdominal wall and pelvic floor concentrically contract just enough to maintain constant pressure. These alternating eccentric and concentric contractions of the abdominal and pelvic floor muscles allow us to breathe and to maintain the proper alignment and load of the spine and legs, which is why I love the hundred exercise. Another example of a sustained load over time is carrying a heavy box or weight for

100 meters (Figure 3-12). The load of the box is constant, and the person will need to maintain the proper load/stiffness relationship while taking numerous breaths over the distance of the 100 meters. Is that person able to breathe naturally and maintain the proper IAP? They should be able to, but there are many who cannot, and you will see them holding their breath or having to take frequent breaks. This is not because they lack strength but because they do not understand the relationship between breath, load, and endurance. They run out of air often by using a Valsalva or breath-holding approach instead of dynamic trunk control in which breathing is easy and sustainable.

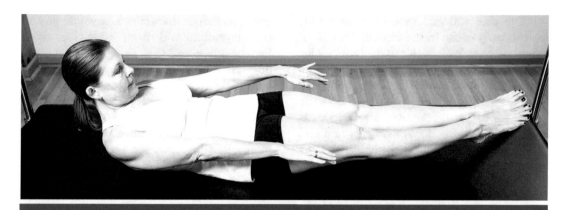

Figure 3-11. The hundred, a breathing and control exercise.

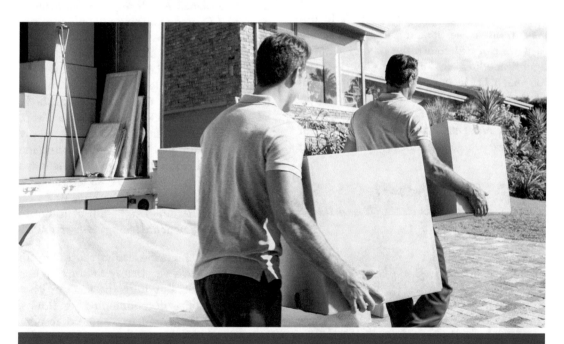

Figure 3-12. Men carrying boxes where prolonged load is constant and requires continuous dynamic control. (KOTOIMAGES/Shutterstock.com.)

PHYSIOLOGY OF BREATH

The physiological control of breath is regulated by chemoreceptors, particularly in our carotid arteries and aorta. These receptors monitor the amount of carbon dioxide (CO_2) in our blood. CO_2 accumulates as a waste product after the body's tissues use the O_2 in the blood. When the levels of CO_2 get high enough, the breathing reflex is triggered.[4] The chemical exchange of O_2 and CO_2 occurs between the alveoli and blood by simple diffusion. O_2 diffuses from the alveoli into the blood and CO_2 from the blood into the alveoli.[4]

The chemical exchange of O_2 and CO_2 gas can only occur in the alveoli. This is an important point because air in the bronchioles (Figure 3-13) does not exchange gases. This may partially explain how free divers and yogis are able to take advantage of holding their breath for up to 10 minutes. This practice is achieved by slowing down the heart rate and redistributing the O_2 within the lungs. There is also another phenomenon in which moisture in the nasal cavity can stimulate an autonomic nervous system reaction that elicits a peripheral vasoconstriction, restricting blood flow from limbs and all organs to preserve blood O_2 for the heart and brain.[18]

Generally, we have plenty of O_2 in our system, but if we breathe more than necessary, we can experience the phenomenon of light-headedness or fainting. When we have too much O_2 in our system from hyperventilation (also called *overbreathing*), the arteries to our brain and other vital organs will constrict, reducing the amount of O_2 to our brain, and we get light-headed. I remember

BRONCHIOLES DO NOT EXCHANGE GAS

ALVEOLI IS WHERE
THE GAS EXCHANGE OCCURS

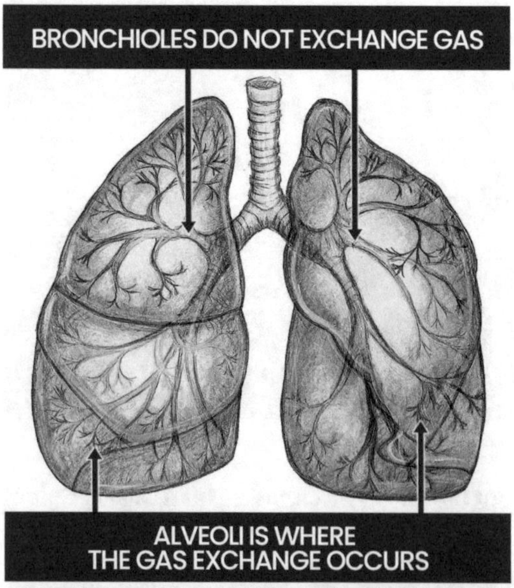

Figure 3-13. The bronchioles and alveoli of the lungs.

(Illustrated by Kelly Anderson.)

trying to induce this effect as a young boy on the playground with my friends. We would hyperventilate and then exhale all the air out one last time as a friend would squeeze us around the chest until we passed out, and a few seconds later we would spontaneously regain consciousness with a little bit of a buzz. Of course, this is not something that I would promote doing now. Have you ever had the experience where you were in a yoga or Pilates class and the instructor was trying to enforce the breath pattern associated with that exercise so much so that when you finished you felt faint or light-headed? In the Polestar vernacular, we often say "Breath is a TOOL not a RULE!" The body is designed to self-regulate the balance between CO_2 and O_2. The body only uses the amount of O_2 that the tissues demand. In yoga, the practice of using less air actually has been shown to increase clarity and alertness.[4,14] In physiology, this is called the *Bohr effect* wherein there is less O_2, or more CO_2, in the body associated with hypoventilation. As a result, vasodilation occurs to increase the O_2 supply to the brain and vital organs, thus increasing alertness and clarity of thought. This leads to the following question: Do we want our clients to breathe for the sake of breathing, or do we want to purposefully use breath as a tool to facilitate movement and energy conservation?

Research shows the leading cause of death in the hospital is respiratory failure.[19] When stale air sits in our lungs because of poor breathing habits, deconditioning, or illness, we have an increased exposure to respiratory infections, especially the resistant strains found in hospitals and long-term care facilities. I have often wondered if we were able to facilitate assisted movement exercises accompanied with breath for patients in acute care, would we minimize the incidence of respiratory failures in these facilities? The internal shower referred to in Joseph Pilates' writings was about taking a few deep inhalations and exhalations per day to cleanse the inner vessels. We can apply the internal shower for the sake of lung hygiene.[5,14]

BIOMECHANICS OF BREATH

The biomechanics of the rib cage and thoracic spine allow for flexibility and movement through many joints, making it possible to breathe in all directions of movement. We have 12 articulating thoracic vertebrae, and each of these movement segments or joints of the spine can move in all planes—flexion, extension, lateral flexion, rotation, translation, and circumduction.[9,20-23]

There are 12 ribs on each side of the spine connecting directly to the transverse process of the corresponding segment. The ribs are the most flexible bone in the body and connect through the sternal costal cartilage (ribs 1 through 7), and the lower ribs (ribs 8 through 10) connect to the 7th rib's costal cartilage; the lower ribs are often referred to as *false ribs*. The 11th and 12th ribs are considered floating ribs and have cartilaginous attachment to the other ribs and, interestingly, have muscular slips that attach to the diaphragm[20,22,23] (Figure 3-14A).

Understanding the biomechanics of the ribs with the spine is essential and often not discussed when talking about breath. We can begin by understanding the anatomical structure of the ribs and how they articulate. The head of each rib articulates with the corresponding vertebra, the intervertebral disc, and the vertebra above[24-28] (Figure 3-14B).

The relationship between the head of the rib and the disc creates the first rule of the ribs—where the disc (or nucleus pulposus [NP]) goes, the rib goes (Figure 3-15). If the vertebral motion segment moves into flexion, the disc will move posteriorly, and by the rule of the ribs, the head of the rib will also glide posteriorly. If the vertebral motion segment moves into extension, then the NP and rib head will move anteriorly. If the motion segment moves into lateral flexion to the right, the NP and both rib heads will translate to the left; the opposite would be true with left lateral flexion,

with the NP and both ribs moving to the right. Rotation typically does not move the disc in any direction; however, the ribs will follow the vertebrae in the direction of rotation.

The second rule of the ribs has to do with the facet on the neck of the rib that articulates with the transverse process of the corresponding vertebra, known as the costovertebral joint (Figure 3-16). At this attachment, when the spine moves into flexion, the rib will move posteriorly, as discussed in the first rule of ribs, and the anterior aspect of the rib will approximate to the rib above. When the segment goes into extension, the NP and the rib head will move anteriorly according to the first rule and will tilt away from the rib of the segment above. Not understanding this rule leads to ineffective cueing and less desirable movement patterns.

The most common faulty movement pattern we observe is the lack of segmental movement in the rib cage. This is often observed in people who play overhead sports (eg, tennis, volleyball, and even swimming) in which spine and rib mobility are especially important. Some people may think they are extending their spine by lifting their chest and visualize the ribs lifting, but they are just extending their low back with a rigid thorax. If all the ribs lift together, then there is no articulation, and the force of the movement is passed down into the lumbar spine or up into the shoulder joint. We want to avoid loading the spine or shoulder at the end of range. If 2 or 3 additional thoracic segments have movement and follow the rule of the ribs, the pressure in the low back and shoulder would greatly decrease. The second rule of the ribs also applies when we move into lateral flexion. If I laterally flex to the right, then both ribs at that segment will translate to the left. The left rib of that segment will tilt down because of its attachment to the inferior transverse process, and the rib on the right will relatively tilt up. This rule facilitates 2 very important principles of the thoracic spine: an increase of axial elongation of the spine and an increase of segmental movement.

[A]
CONNECTIVE TISSUE

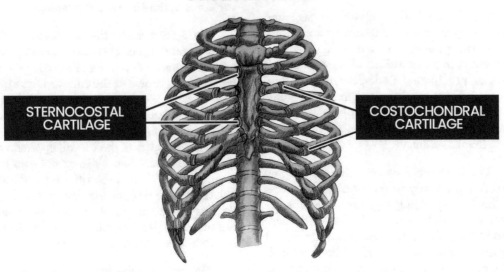

STERNOCOSTAL CARTILAGE

COSTOCHONDRAL CARTILAGE

[B]
COSTOVERTEBRAL AND COSTOTRANSVERSE JOINTS

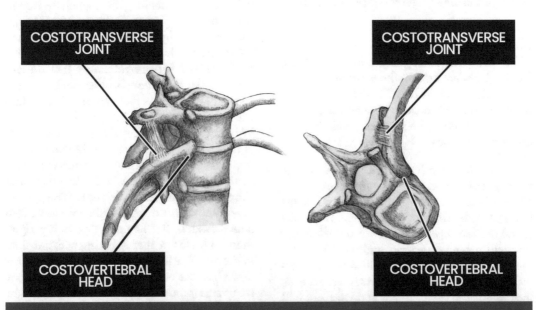

COSTOTRANSVERSE JOINT

COSTOTRANSVERSE JOINT

COSTOVERTEBRAL HEAD

COSTOVERTEBRAL HEAD

Figure 3-14. (A) Connective tissue and (B) joints of the rib cage.

(Illustrated by Kelly Anderson.)

The last movement plane with the second rule of the ribs is rotation. We need to rely on another biomechanical rule from Harrison Fryette, which states that in the lower thoracic and lumbar spine, the vertebrae of a motion segment will rotate and laterally flex in opposite directions.[28] If we look at the L3-4 motion segment and side bend to the right, the segment will naturally tend to rotate to the left. The same thing happens in the thorax. Often in Pilates and yoga, we think about rotation as if it happens without this movement coupling. Therefore, when we are rotating, we must axially elongate the spine to optimize movement in the desired direction (ie, rotation) and minimize movement in the unwanted direction (ie, lateral flexion).

Many will experience a significant increase in total rotation with greater ease just by applying the image of the rule of the ribs. Golfers and tennis players will pay a lot of money for this information.

As I mentioned previously, a common faulty movement strategy is to move too much in the lumbar spine, especially at L4-L5-S1. Increasing the segmental movements of the spine, even in 2 to 3 new segments in the upper lumbar and thoracic spine, can significantly reduce the excessive force transmitted through the lumbar spine. Over time, the excessive force and repetition of moving in a limited number of segments can lead to overuse and degenerative changes. Improved spinal mobility is probably one of the greatest benefits of practicing Pilates, yoga, Gyrotonic Expansion System, Feldenkrais Method, and other mindful movement training programs. Each of these movement forms focus on 3-dimensional breath strategies resulting in improved spine mobility. Theoretically, increasing the availability of controlled movement options throughout the spine and joints of the extremities should reduce undesirable excessive forces experienced when only a few joints are bearing the load. This distribution of movement can minimize unwanted or excessive forces passing through the lumbar, thoracic, and cervical spine, as well as the shoulders and hips,

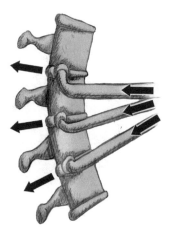

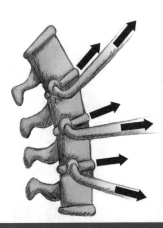

Figure 3-15. The first rule of the ribs.
(Illustrated by Kelly Anderson.)

and improve motor learning options to execute daily tasks. This is discussed in much greater depth in Chapter 4.

When we look at the nature of the movement of ribs, the first 7 ribs, which are called *true ribs*, have a rotational bias within the facet of the transverse process of the vertebrae below.[20,23] In ribs 8 through 10, the facets of the ribs are more planar and have a gliding bias that expands the rib cage laterally. Notice that I use the word bias because all the ribs are capable of both the rotation that facilitates an anterior expansion of the rib cage and a lateral glide, which facilitates lateral expansion of the

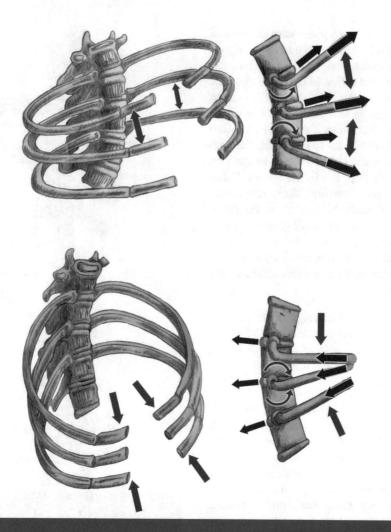

Figure 3-16. The second rule of ribs as seen in extension above and flexion below. (Illustrated by Kelly Anderson.)

rib cage (Figure 3-17). Even though each joint can rotate and glide laterally, the tendency is to have more anterior chest displacement from the upper ribs, which is often compared to the handle of an old-fashioned water pump (Figure 3-18A). Lateral chest displacement from the lower ribs can be compared to a bucket handle (Figure 3-18B).[9,21,29]

Remember that during breath, movement occurs in all 3 planes: vertical (up and down), coronal (right and left), and sagittal (front and back). We can start by understanding the superior and inferior dimension of the rib cage. When we breathe, the diaphragm contracts, and the lungs and lower rib cage expand inferiorly and forward because of the angulation of the attachment to the lower ribs. The superior vertical displacement occurs when we use accessory breathing muscles to lift the ribs (Figure 3-19). Accessory breathing, as mentioned previously, is not the most efficient way to breathe and is often associated with faulty breathing habits because of the amount of work needed to lift the ribs compared with other forms of efficient air exchange. Lateral expansion of the rib cage occurs in the coronal plane with ribs 8 through 10 and is often called *bucket handle breathing*. However, lateral expansion is not limited to ribs 8 through 10. For example, if you were to put your right hand behind your head and side bend to the left, you would notice that most of the movement occurs in the lower rib cage; however, you will notice that there is movement in the upper ribs as well. This movement can further be enhanced by directing the breath into the upper portion of the right lung and applying the image of the second rule of the ribs. Finally, expansion anteriorly and posteriorly or in the sagittal plane can be most noticeable in the upper chest. Typically, we expand the ribs more anteriorly than posteriorly, but it is important to note that the rib cage and vertebra can expand posteriorly. This breath pattern is often associated with flexion of the thoracic spine; likewise, anterior displacement of the rib cage is often associated with extension of the thoracic spine. The greater the suppleness and options of movement in the thorax, the more likely movement and breath can be spontaneous, fluid, and automatic.

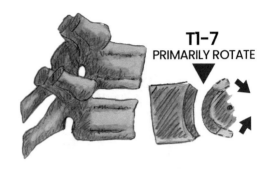

T1-7
PRIMARILY ROTATE

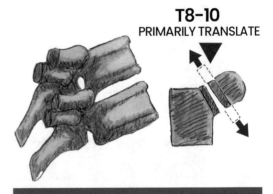

T8-10
PRIMARILY TRANSLATE

Figure 3-17. The transverse costal facet.
(Illustrated by Kelly Anderson.)

[A]
WATER PUMP HANDLE MECHANICS IS EQUATED TO ANTERIOR DISPLACEMENT OF STERNUM AND RIB CAGE

[B]
BUCKET HANDLE MECHANICS IS EQUATED TO LATERAL DISPLACEMENT OF THE RIB CAGE

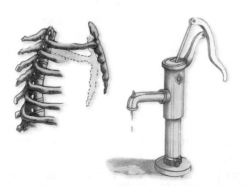
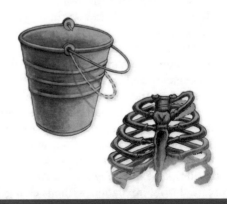

Figure 3-18. The (A) water pump handle and (B) bucket handle.
(Illustrated by Kelly Anderson.)

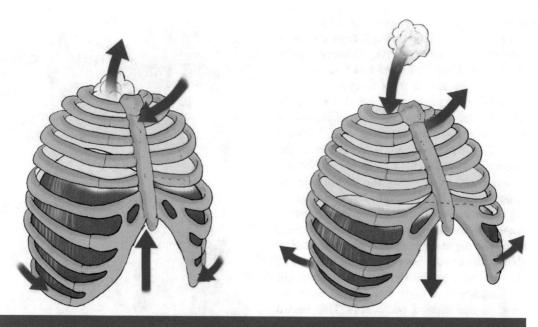

Figure 3-19. Exhale and inhale in 3 dimensions.

APPLICATION
MOTOR CONTROL

Most air exchange in the lungs occurs from the contraction of the diaphragm. As we explored earlier, the domes of the diaphragm are attached through the central tendon to the pleura of the lungs. When the muscle fibers contract, they draw the central tendon inferiorly and anteriorly based on the angle of the diaphragm, which flattens the diaphragm, decreasing the pressure in the lungs and facilitating inhalation. You should notice that the abdomen expands and relaxes in response to the movement of the diaphragm. Therefore, the abdominal wall is important for healthy breathing, IAP regulation, and spine control in combination with the pelvic floor and diaphragm. They must have a dynamic relationship that allows the diaphragm to expand into the viscera during inhalation without changing the IAP. Ideally, this results in an eccentric contraction of the abdominal wall and pelvic floor while the diaphragm is concentrically

contracting and compressing the viscera. Exhalation is the relaxation of the diaphragm and its return to its resting position because of elastic memory. The amount of eccentric and concentric contraction depends on the type of movement, the load of an activity, and how much IAP is required to perform that task successfully. Also taken into consideration is the respiratory demand based on the workload of the body during an activity. If forced inhalation or exhalation is required, the abdominal, pelvic floor, and intercostal muscles will respond appropriately to maintain the proper IAP needed based on the anticipated load of the task at hand.

I have had many patients and clients refer to themselves as "bad breathers." When I asked them who had told them they were bad breathers, they often responded that it was their therapist, personal trainer, Pilates, or yoga teacher. This is very interesting when we consider that these people are in key positions of authority, and what they say can have great influence on their clients' perception of themselves. Perception can influence outcome as much as 80%,[30] and it is necessary we create positive images and remember that clients and patients take to heart what we say. After all, what good comes from telling someone they are bad at something? When a client or patient tells me they are a bad breather, I often say that is impossible. Why? Because every bad breather I know is dead. Can we learn to breathe more efficiently and increase our functional breath capacity? The answer is a resounding yes!

Clients and patients often have a bias to a particular breath pattern. We can use movement to facilitate breathing patterns that are challenging, especially regions of the thorax that are particularly limited. Body position can greatly influence where breath will occur. For example, the child's pose can facilitate breath into the posterior aspect of the thorax and improve the breath capacity in the anterior-posterior dimension. I can also position someone who is primarily an accessory breather in seated spinal flexion. By lowering the head into flexion, this removes the ability to use an accessory breath strategy. I then ask them to start to breathe deeply, which may cause a sense of panic because they have to find another breath strategy, but 9 of 10 times they will rediscover an old, more efficient breathing pattern by using the diaphragm or expanding the inferior rib cage. Clients might feel very uncomfortable when you make a change to their breathing pattern, so be patient and allow them to adjust their position if needed. It may take time to be able to move the rib cage and find mobility in the spine, but with consistent practice, the patterns will change and breathing will become less effortful and more efficient. A skilled and kind teacher will help clients find new breathing strategies in different physical postures guided by proper instruction. We do not want anyone to pass out or feel terribly uncomfortable, so remember to use movement and positioning to improve breathing efficiency and capacity that is client-centric.

From a movement science perspective, we often say "breath facilitates movement and movement facilitates breath." How do we understand the principle of breath in a way that we can optimize the appropriate amount of expansion and contraction of the rib cage and diaphragm so that it naturally, efficiently, and spontaneously matches the demand of the desired movement or task? This is the most important question because complex movement requires the ability to breathe spontaneously.[3] Imagine playing tennis or volleyball and insisting that inhalation occurs every time the spine moves into extension and exhalation occurs every time the body moves into flexion. You would not be able to play. This is a common mistake when teaching basic exercises. We often hyperventilate our clients by telling them to always exhale on exertion even if the exertion is not that strong, or tell them they must inhale or exhale at a particular time in the movement. Can our clients choose the opposite breath pattern and exhale with extension and inhale with flexion or other combined movements? Of course they can. This reinforces the following statement: "Breath is a tool not a rule." Our ideal objective is to make sure that our clients can breathe in all planes and in all positions.

So, what would restrict or limit a client's ability to breathe in all dimensions? It could be their movement strategy, in that they have mobility in all directions but do not have the awareness or training to organize their body efficiently. Others might have a real structural restriction that requires structural intervention, such as fascial release, joint mobilization, and even surgery in some extreme situations. What causes structural restrictions? Structural restrictions may result from a congenital postural deviation, such as scoliosis or scar tissue from surgery, radiation, or an injury.[31] Restrictions can also result from chronic poor posture. In myofascial science, the dynamic fascial organ that connects to all nonfluid cells in the body is always remodeling itself. It can be thought of as a 3-dimensional printer that is continually printing the fascia in 3 dimensions according to the loads applied to the tissue.[13] If we have poor postural habits for prolonged periods of time, our fascial organ, which is thought by some research to be present in every nonfluid cell, including cartilage, bone, discs, and ligaments, will take a new shape. Even just sitting for too long at the movies makes it hard to stand up straight for a couple minutes. Eric Franklin said, "We are what we practice."[32] What are you practicing?

Another consideration with breathing is whether breath interferes with or facilitates the quality of movement. Three common movement or postural faults that we see are as follows:

1. Accessory breathing: As we have already explored, accessory breathing is typically the result of poor posture, smoking, and COPD. A slouched posture with rounded shoulders and a forward head creates the perfect storm in which the only breath option is to use accessory breathing muscles because the slouched position limits movement of the diaphragm and abdominal wall (Figure 3-20). It is important to remember that accessory breathing can be used to complement maximum breath capacity in endurance activities, compromised structural posture issues, or systemic breathing diseases, such as asthma or COPD.

2. Flared rib cage: Obesity, pregnancy, and loss of connectivity between the thorax and pelvis as we age are often the culprits of a flared rib cage. A flared rib cage can arise from a lack of tensile forces between the inferior ribs and the superior rim of the pelvis. The tension or tensegrity is a result of a healthy relationship of the abdominal and back myofascial connections. The myofascial connections help to align the rib cage with the pelvis, provide the essential elasticity, and allow for proper force distribution throughout the body during our normal, varied daily movement tasks. In a flared rib cage, instead of the ribs being angled downward, the ribs will elevate to a more horizontal orientation and

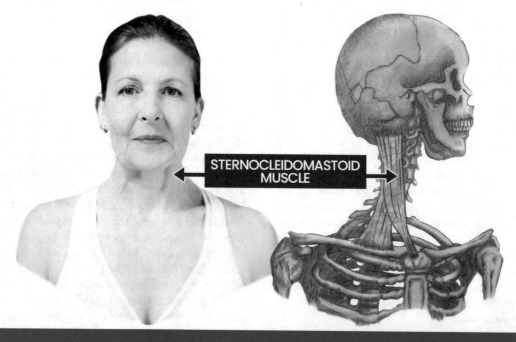

STERNOCLEIDOMASTOID MUSCLE

Figure 3-20. Accessory breathing.

lose their alignment with the pelvis. We can use an example of a tube or cylinder in which the diameter of the tube is the same as the diameter of the thorax and pelvis (Figure 3-21A). Our goal is to create a relationship of equal circumference comparatively between the torso and the pelvis. In the example of a flared rib cage, the thorax has a much greater circumference than the pelvic rim (Figure 3-21B). Instead of a tube from the thorax to the pelvis, it would look more like a funnel, with the wider opening at the bottom of the ribs. Imagine how this affects breath capacity and potentially increases the risk of respiratory disease because of less circulation in the inferior lobes of the lungs. When the lower rib cage is flared and limited in its ability to narrow, the lower lobes of the lungs will be full of stale air. There is no way to push the air out. This is common postpartum for women and is often observed with obesity. The ideal

angle of the xiphoid process to the lower ribs should be approximately 90 degrees, whereas a flared rib cage can be as much as 180 degrees (Figures 3-22A and 3-22B).

3. Mechanical insufficiency of the diaphragm: Many fitness enthusiasts misunderstand the role of the abdominal muscles. Instead of a dynamic abdominal wall to efficiently manage IAP, they create a situation in which the abdominal muscles are over-recruited for aesthetic reasons (ie, "look at my 6-pack"), resulting in abdominal contractures (overly tight and restricted abdominal muscles). When the muscles stay in this contracted state for extended periods of time and a contracture of the anterior abdominal wall occurs, the muscles can no longer lengthen eccentrically. This leaves little room for the viscera to expand. When the diaphragm is too restricted, it often becomes actively insufficient and unable to descend or expand, resulting in other

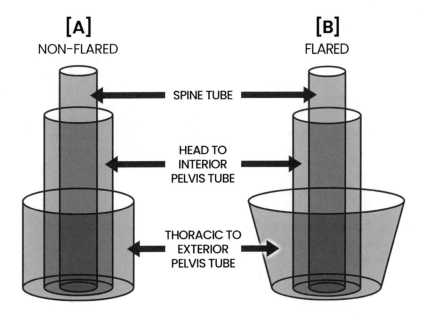

DR. BRENT ANDERSON'S TUBULAR MODEL OF THE TRUNK © 2023

Figure 3-21. Three tubes: (A) nonflared and (B) flared. (Illustrated by Kelly Anderson.)

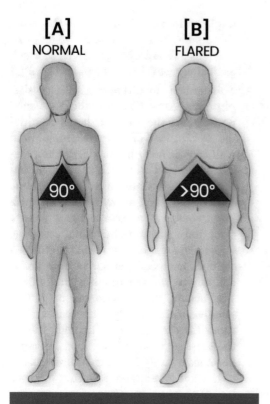

[A]
NORMAL

[B]
FLARED

90°

>90°

Figure 3-22. (A) Normal and (B) flared rib cage.   (Illustrated by Kelly Anderson.)

Prana is the energy that drives life, the power that animates the body, enlivens the mind, spurs the soul. Prana is life's inspiration, its foundation, its tenacity; it is the sure hand on the tiller, the wise voice of good counsel, the urge to health and harmony that craves to turn our bodies into havens where we can take shelter from the storms of the hectic modern world. Prana is at work at every instant in every cell of every living organism.[33]

PRACTICAL APPLICATIONS OF BREATH

Breath can be used to facilitate and to resist all directions of movement. Remember that the direction of breath is always related to the 3-dimensional displacement of the rib cage and the diaphragm.

MOBILITY

Inhalation into the upper rib cage facilitates spine extension, and inhalation into the lower rib cage facilitates spine flexion, especially when the spine is already biased toward flexion. Exhalation primarily facilitates spine flexion; unilateral exhalation facilitates lateral flexion to the same side. Breath into one lung influences lateral flexion of the rib cage and spine.

compensatory breath strategies. This faulty movement strategy is opposite of the flared rib cage in which the inferior xyphoid angle is now less than 90 degrees.

BIOENERGETICS

According to Robert Edwin Svoboda, "Breath, prana, and mind are mutually and inherently related; cultivate one well and the other two will fall into line."[33] He also stated the following:

STABILITY

Exhalation using the abdominal wall will resist the tendency for the spine to extend when the extremities are moving away from the body. Inhalation can be used to resist the tendency to flex the spine when the extremities are moving toward the center of the body (Figures 3-23A and 3-23B).

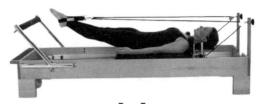

[A]
LEGS AWAY FROM THE BODY

GENERATE FORCE

Forced exhalation can increase IAP, narrow the rib cage, and increase the stability of the trunk while exerting forces, such as kicking, lifting, and swinging. The tendency in learning a new movement is to over-recruit, thus losing efficiency of breath, which is necessary with complex movements. The more efficient and coordinated the breath and movement are, the more productive the force will be; in other words, you will hit the ball farther.

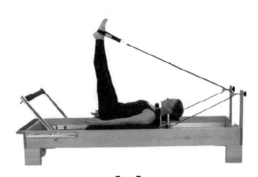

[B]
LEGS TOWARD THE BODY

Figure 3-23. Feet in straps exercise on reformer: (A) legs away from the body and (B) legs toward the body.

OPEN-ENDED QUESTIONS

1 Describe in your own words the 3 mechanical dimensions of breath. How might breath direction bias affect spine movement? Give an example.

2 Explain how the contraction of the diaphragm influences movement and internal pressure of the lungs.

3 Draw a diagram of the crura of the diaphragm and show how it crosses the apex of the lumbar spine. What relevance might this play pertaining to control of the trunk?

4 Describe in your own words how the abdominal muscles, diaphragm, and intercostal and back muscles influence the increase and decrease of IAP. How does this relate to the hydraulic amplifier?

OPEN-ENDED QUESTIONS

5   Explain how a Valsalva breath technique could interfere with normal movement. How should IAP be maintained if not by holding one's breath or volitionally contracting abdominal muscles?

6   How do the pubococcygeus and the diaphragm work together? Anatomically, what do they share?

7   Describe the difference between subconscious and submaximal contractions and max voluntary contractions.

8   List muscle groups responsible for moving the rib cage/lungs.

9   What movement or control is achieved by the same muscles of breath?

10   Describe in your own words the first rule of the ribs and how it relates to movement in each direction.

11   Describe in your own words the second rule of the ribs and how it can relate to movement in each direction.

12   Explain the biomechanics/movement of ribs 1 through 7 during inhalation, also known as the "water pump mechanism."

13   Explain the biomechanics/movement of ribs 8 through 10 during inhalation, also referred to as the "bucket handle" motion.

14   Expand on the rule of ribs and biomechanical properties of the costovertebral joints and how they might facilitate multidirectional movements (ie, a golf swing).

15   Explain how the vocal cords, diaphragm, and pelvic floor theoretically assist in upright posture.

16   How might the hundred exercise described in the chapter and carrying a heavy box 100 m have similarities? How do breath and control relate to each other?

17   What is your breathing bias and how does it compare to that of a companion or partner?

18   Differentiate how a structural restriction could affect movement quality vs how a strategic restriction might affect the quality of movement.

OPEN-ENDED QUESTIONS

19 How would you describe a healthy relationship between the circumference of the thorax and the pelvis?

20 How might the strategy to have "a 6-pack" abdominal wall interfere with normal diaphragmatic movement? Describe how it might influence IAP.

21 Discuss how breath can be used to facilitate mobility and control/stability, generate force, and for relaxation.

22 Explain the energetic concepts of breath as they integrate with anatomy, physiology, and movement science. What lessons can we learn and teach to our clients regarding breath's effect on perception, belief, and spirit?

REFERENCES

1. Genesis 2:7 (KJV).
2. Morgan BJ, Crabtree DC, Palta M, Skatrud JB. Combined hypoxia and hypercapnia evokes long-lasting sympathetic activation in humans. *J Appl Physiol (1985)*. 1995;79(1):205-213.
3. Calais-Germain B. *Anatomy of Breathing*. Eastland Press; 2006.
4. Borg-Olivier S. *Applied Anatomy & Physiology of Yoga*. Warisanoffset.com; 2006.
5. Pilates JH, Miller WJ, Robbins J, Van Heuit-Robbins L. *Pilates Evolution: The 21st Century*. Presentation Dynamics; 2012.
6. Pilates JH. *Return to Life Through Contrology*. J. J. Augustin Publisher; 1945.
7. Craighero S, Promayon E, Baconnier P, Lebas JF, Coulomb M. Dynamic echo-planar MR imaging of the diaphragm for a 3D dynamic analysis. *Eur Radiol*. 2005;15(4):742-748.
8. Williams PL, Warwick R, eds. *Gray's Anatomy*. Churchill Livingston; 1980.
9. Harrison DE, Jones EW, Janik TJ, Harrison DD. Evaluation of axial and flexural stresses in the vertebral body cortex and trabecular bone in lordosis and two sagittal cervical translation configurations with an elliptical shell model. *J Manipulative Physiol Ther*. 2002;25(6):391-401.
10. Kolar P, Sulc J, Kyncl M, et al. Postural function of the diaphragm in persons with and without chronic low back pain. *J Orthop Sports Phys Ther*. 2012;42(4):352-362.
11. Hodges PW, Cresswell AG, Daggfeldt K, Thorstensson A. In vivo measurement of the effect of intra-abdominal pressure on the human spine. *J Biomech*. 2001;34(3):347-353.
12. Norris C. Spinal stabilisation, 1. Active lumbar stabilisation–2. Limiting factors to end-range of motion in the lumbar spine–3. Stabilisation mechanisms of the lumbar spine. *Physiother J*. 1995;81(2):61-79.
13. Lederman E. The fall of the postural-structural-biomechanical model in manual and physical therapies: exemplified by lower back pain. *J Bodyw Mov Ther*. 2011;15(2):131-138.
14. Hewitt J. *The Complete Yoga Book: Yoga of Breathing, Yoga of Posture, and Yoga of Meditation*. Schocken Books; 1978.
15. Massery M, Hagins M, Stafford R, Moerchen V, Hodges PW. Effect of airway control by glottal structures on postural stability. *J Appl Physiol*. 2013;115(4):483-490.
16. Hodges PW, Richardson CA. Inefficient muscular stabilization of the lumbar spine associated with low back pain: a motor control evaluation of transversus abdominis. *Spine*. 1996;21(22):2640-2650.
17. McGill S. *Low Back Disorders: Evidence-Based Prevention and Rehabilitation*. 2nd ed. Human Kinetics; 2007.
18. Bosco G, Rizzato A, Martani L, et al. Arterial blood gas analysis in breath-hold divers at depth. *Front Physiol*. 2018;9:1558.
19. CDC/NCHS. National Hospital Discharge Survey. 2000, 2005, 2010.

20. Harrison DE, Cailliet R, Harrison DD, Janik TJ. How do anterior/posterior translations of the thoracic cage affect the sagittal lumbar spine, pelvic tilt, and thoracic kyphosis? *Eur Spine J.* 2002;11(3):287-293.

21. Harrison DE, Colloca CJ, Harrison DD, Janik TJ, Haas JW, Keller TS. Anterior thoracic posture increases thoracolumbar disc loading. *Eur Spine J.* 2005;14(3):234-242.

22. Lee D, Delta Orthopaedic Physiotherapy Clinic. *Manual Therapy for the Thorax: A Biomechanical Approach.* DOPC; 1994.

23. Tsang SM, Szeto GP, Lee RY. Normal kinematics of the neck: the interplay between the cervical and thoracic spines. *Man Ther.* 2013;18(5):431-437.

24. Dickey JP, Kerr DJ. Effect of specimen length: are the mechanics of individual motion segments comparable in functional spinal units and multisegment specimens? *Med Eng Phys.* 2003;25(3):221-227.

25. Saker E, Graham RA, Nicholas R, et al. Ligaments of the costovertebral joints including biomechanics, innervations, and clinical applications: a comprehensive review with application to approaches to the thoracic spine. *Cureus.* 2016;8(11):e874.

26. Beyer B, Sholukha V, Dugailly PM, et al. In vivo thorax 3D modelling from costovertebral joint complex kinematics. *Clin Biomech (Bristol, Avon).* 2014;29(4):434-438.

27. Lee DG. Biomechanics of the thorax - research evidence and clinical expertise. *J Man Manip Ther.* 2015;23(3):128-138.

28. Bayliss J. Spinal mechanics. 2005. http://spinalmechanics.com/fryette.html

29. Harrison DE, Janik TJ, Cailliet R, et al. Upright static pelvic posture as rotations and translations in 3-dimensional from three 2-dimensional digital images: validation of a computerized analysis. *J Manipulative Physiol Ther.* 2008;31(2):137-145.

30. Lackner JM, Carosella AM. The relative influence of perceived pain control, anxiety, and functional self efficacy on spinal function among patients with chronic low back pain. *Spine (Phila Pa 1976).* 1999;24(21):2254-2260; discussion 2260-2251.

31. Lee KJ, Roper JG, Wang JC. Demineralized bone matrix and spinal arthrodesis. *Spine J.* 2005;5(suppl):217S-223S.

32. Franklin EN. *Conditioning for Dance.* Human Kinetics; 2004.

33. Svoboda RE. Cultivating prana. 2000. https://drsvoboda.com/articles/ayurveda/cultivating-prana/

MOBILITY

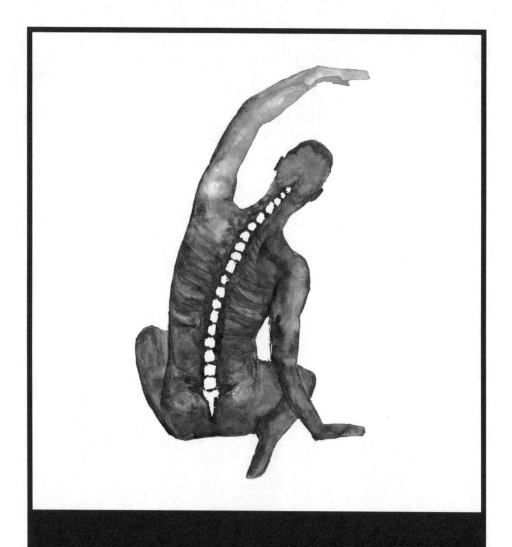

THE DISTRIBUTION OF MOVEMENT EQUALS THE DISTRIBUTION OF FORCE.

CHAPTER 4

CHAPTER OBJECTIVES

1 Understand how mobility directly influences movement efficiency and function.

2 Define the different properties of movement related to the different structure and orientations of the cervical, thoracic, and lumbar spine.

3 Comprehend the neuromuscular system's effect on joint mobility and control.

4 Apply biomechanics of the axial skeleton and the extremities to acquisition and/or restoration of functional movement.

5 Differentiate between osteokinematics and arthrokinematics, and identify how to observe abilities and restrictions of both.

6 Apply the biomechanical properties of the upper and lower extremities and their integration into trunk movement.

KEY TERMS
- Arthrokinematics
- Articulation
- Axial elongation
- Bandha
- Bone rhythms
- Glide
- Global muscles
- Local muscles
- Mobility
- Noncontractile
- Spin
- Spiral

Mobility is necessary before control. Before someone can have control, they need to have mobility; otherwise, what are they controlling? Stability is the control of mobility. I have taught movement for more than 30 years, and I never cease to be impressed with the power associated with restoring mobility to the human body. Mobility must be present before the neuromuscular system can control it. Without mobility, we are rigid, and our movement options are limited. Clinically, I have found that a large percentage of what look like structural movement restrictions turn out to be strategic restrictions. In this chapter, we will learn to differentiate between structural and strategic movement restrictions. The

more efficient a practitioner becomes at differentiating between structure and strategy, the more effective they will become at restoring functional movement and minimizing potentially harmful forces.

THE DISTRIBUTION OF MOVEMENT EQUALS THE DISTRIBUTION OF FORCE.

The key focus in this chapter is the distribution of movement equals the distribution of force. Basically, this means that by efficiently moving from more segments, a person can potentially reduce the stress to the surrounding joints that often leads to pathology and degeneration. Joseph Pilates said, "If your

Anderson BD.
Principles of Movement (pp 56-96).
© 2024 Taylor & Francis Group.

spine is inflexibly stiff at 30, you are old. If it is completely flexible at 60, you are young."[1] What great insight that our bodies can be made young or old merely by the amount of flexibility or suppleness in our spine. As a physical therapist, I see this all the time. I have clients in their 80s who are young because they have made mobility activities a priority in their lives. A client with knee pain will do better if their lower extremity strategy focuses on hip and ankle mobility rather than solely focusing on mobility of the knee. Mobility in neighboring joints to reduce the load in painful or pathological joints is a worthy strategy. It often results in directly decreasing the stress in the painful or injured joint while increasing function. On numerous occasions, simply changing the strategy of a squat, reach, or lift activity to the surrounding joints can be enough to eliminate the joint stress being interpreted as pain.

ESSENTIAL SCIENCES
AXIAL SKELETON MOBILITY: BONES OF THE SPINE

I love teaching movement from the bones. To do this, it is essential that we wholly understand the anatomy and biomechanics of the skeleton and joints. Let us start with the amazing anatomy of the spine. The spine can be divided into 4 sections. The first one is the sacrum or the base of the spine (Figures 4-1A and 4-1B). It is a triangular-shaped bone that is made up of smaller fused segments. The sacrum is connected to the pelvis through a series of thick and strong ligaments both posteriorly and anteriorly (Figures 4-2A and 4-2B). There is not a lot of movement that occurs between the sacrum and the pelvis.[2] The pelvis is made up of 2 large bones called the *ilia*, which are often referred to as the *innominate bones*. The innominate bones articulate posteriorly, with the sacrum making up the sacroiliac joints (SIJ). The fronts of the innominate

[A]
ANTERIOR VIEW OF SACRUM

[B]
POSTERIOR VIEW OF SACRUM

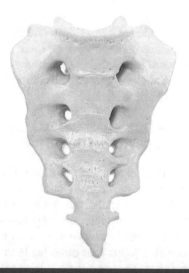
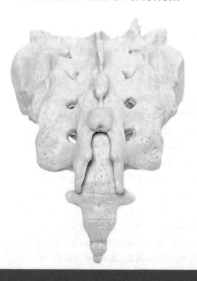

Figure 4-1. The sacrum. (A) The anterior view of the sacrum. (B) The posterior view of the sacrum.

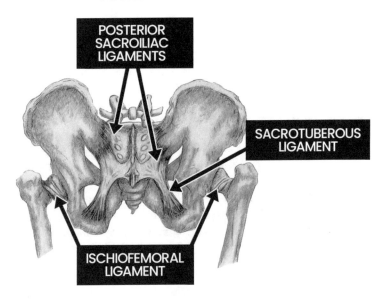

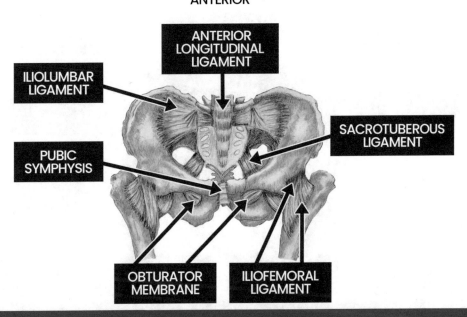

Figure 4-2. The (A) posterior and (B) anterior SIJ ligaments. (Illustrated by Kelly Anderson.)

bones articulate together through the pubic rami with the pubic disk in between them to make up the pubic symphysis (Figure 4-3).

The lumbopelvic region, including the SIJ, is thought by many to be the origin or center of movement. The SIJ is made to absorb force and release potential energy as we move. There is much controversy regarding the movement of the SIJ. Manual therapies often assume that the SIJ possesses small amounts of movement; it can flair, spin, and twist. Conversely, most anatomists believe that there is no movement in the SIJ. For the purpose of this book, I will compromise between the 2 schools of SIJ mobility, and we will assume that the SIJ absorbs and releases the ground reaction forces between the lower extremities and the spine.

The spine consists of 24 vertebrae and 23 intervertebral disks (Figure 4-4). Directly above the sacrum are 5 vertebrae called the *lumbar vertebrae* (Figure 4-5). They are primarily designed to bear weight, and their bodies are vertical and stocky. The facets align in a

vertical orientation and move in the sagittal plane (flexion and extension or forward and back bending). In addition to flexion and extension, the lumbar spine has a moderate amount of lateral flexion and very little rotation.[3-6]

The next grouping of vertebrae comprises the thoracic spine. There are 12 ribs on each side attaching to the 12 thoracic vertebrae (Figure 4-6). The thoracic facets have a coronal orientation of about 65 degrees and are designed to facilitate rotation more than lateral flexion.[7-10] The thoracic spine plays a significant role in improving the dexterity of the upper extremities and the head.[2,3,10-13] This part of our body is meant to protect the vital organs within the thorax. We do not often think about the thorax when thinking about the arms, but the ribs and thoracic spine have a direct impact on the quality of the movement in the upper extremity.

If we were to perform an experiment by taking away our thoracic mobility by slouching and then attempt to turn our head side

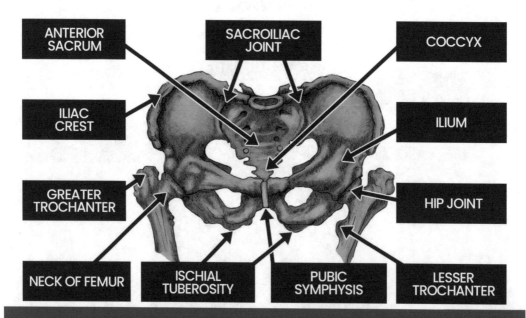

ANTERIOR SACRUM

SACROILIAC JOINT

COCCYX

ILIAC CREST

ILIUM

GREATER TROCHANTER

HIP JOINT

NECK OF FEMUR

ISCHIAL TUBEROSITY

PUBIC SYMPHYSIS

LESSER TROCHANTER

Figure 4-3. The anterior SIJ and the pubic symphysis.   (Illustrated by Kelly Anderson.)

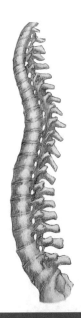

Figure 4-4. The spine.
(Illustrated by Kelly Anderson.)

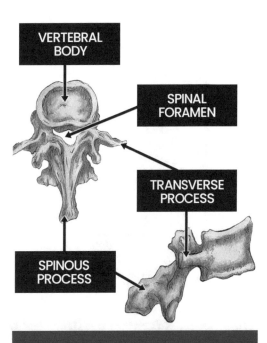

Figure 4-5. The lumbar spine.
(Illustrated by Kelly Anderson.)

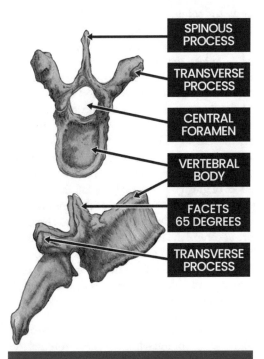

SPINOUS PROCESS

TRANSVERSE PROCESS

CENTRAL FORAMEN

VERTEBRAL BODY

FACETS 65 DEGREES

TRANSVERSE PROCESS

Figure 4-6. The thoracic spine.
(Illustrated by Kelly Anderson.)

to side or raise our arms above our head, we would observe that both movements are limited and possibly uncomfortable. If we allow our rib cage to assume a more vertical posture and turn our head or raise our arms, we will observe much greater range of motion and more comfort. Observe a tennis player serving or a pitcher throwing a baseball. The thorax, head, shoulders, and arms work in harmony to both create and distribute force and movement. If they did not, the shoulder would most probably take the brunt of the force.

The cervical spine is made up of 7 segments (Figure 4-7). It has the greatest degrees of freedom of all the segments of the spine. The cervical spine gives the head mobility so that we can access our senses, most importantly, our vision and hearing. The vertebrae C3-7 have an orientation of approximately 45 degrees, whereas the upper 2 vertebrae, C1 and C2, and the head have a horizontal orientation (Figure 4-8). They are responsible for upwards of 50% of the head's movement in rotation and side bending.

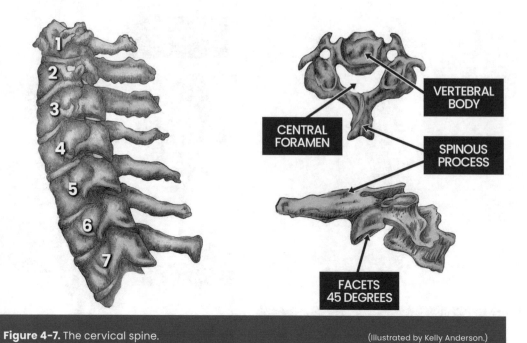

Figure 4-7. The cervical spine.   (Illustrated by Kelly Anderson.)

MUSCLES OF THE SPINE

Attached to the bones in the head, thorax, pelvis, and the spine are many muscles that facilitate movement and support of the axial skeleton. We often think of them in 2 groups, global and superficial or local and deep. Following is a quick review of global vs local muscle function. Global muscles can be defined as muscles that when they contract generate directional movement.[14] They can either accelerate or decelerate the body's movement. When we talk about global muscles of the trunk, we often refer to muscles such as the rectus abdominis, the external obliques and internal obliques at the front of the body (Figure 4-9; see Figure 3-7B in Chapter 3), the quadratus lumborum (QL), and the longissimus thoracis and iliocostalis lumborum (part of the erector spinae muscle group in the back; Figure 4-10). These large muscles cover a span of multiple segments of the spine, some bypassing tendinous insertions into the lumbar spine with insertions in the pelvis and thorax. Bypassing insertion of these global muscles into the pelvis can create compressive and shear forces in the lumbar spine if not countered with

local stiffening around the lumbar segments themselves. When the global muscles contract, they create forces that can rotate, extend, flex, or compress the spine. If I were lying on my back and wanted to sit up, I could concentrically contract my rectus abdominis to flex my spine. These muscles also work eccentrically (lengthening with control) and slow down or decelerate movement. If I were to bend forward while standing, my spine extensors, the erector spinae, would work eccentrically to help control the effect of gravity so I would not fall forward. If I were going into a backbend from a standing position, my rectus abdominis would eccentrically fire to control the movement of my spine into the backbend. We refer to the muscles functionally as *global mobilizers* if they are concentrically contracting and *global stabilizers* if they are eccentrically contracting.[2,15,16]

The second grouping of muscles are the local or deep muscles.[14] These muscles do not have a direction of movement per se and typically provide a stiffening or cocontraction around the spinal joints. These local muscles allow for segmental articulation of the spine.

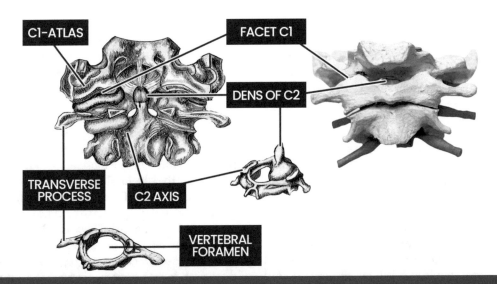

Figure 4-8. C1-2.

(Illustrated by Kelly Anderson.)

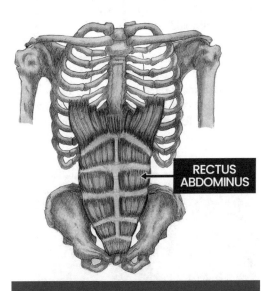

Figure 4-9. The rectus abdominis.

(Illustrated by Kelly Anderson.)

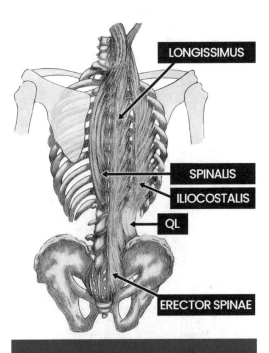

Figure 4-10. The superficial muscles of the back.

(Illustrated by Kelly Anderson.)

Muscles in one area of the spine can stiffen, which allows the vertebra above or below to move. We often refer to the cocontraction of these muscles as a *force couple*, or in yoga, a *bandha*. They work subconsciously to prepare the body for movement of the limbs or the torso.[14,17] They create the appropriate amount of stiffness for an anticipated load.[18,19] This means they will contract more or less depending on the movement or task. You would not want to use the same strategy or level of local stiffness to pick up a heavy box as you would a set of keys off the floor.

This deep muscle group includes the transverse abdominis, internal obliques (see Figure 3-7), pelvic floor complex muscles (see Figure 3-9), multifidi (Figure 4-11), medial fibers of the QL and psoas major (Figure 4-12), longissimus thoracis, and iliocostalis lumborum (see Figure 4-10). You will notice that some muscles can fit into both categories (ie, global and local stabilizers). Which category they fall into depends on the proximity of the fibers to the spine and how many segments they affect, typically within 2 to 5 segments. Often the shorter fibers found closest to the spine act more as stiffening muscles rather than movement muscles. For example, the psoas major muscle (see Figure 4-12) flexes the hip

and is considered a global muscle; however, the superior medial fibers of the psoas major attach to the spine traversing 2 to 4 vertebral segments[3,20-22] and provide anterolateral stiffening, as a local muscle, to the lower thoracic and upper lumbar vertebrae.

These small muscles connect and provide feedback to the central nervous system through high concentrations of muscle spindle fibers. We can say that the local muscles, or deep local stabilizers', primary function is to provide proprioception and stiffness to the joint complexes appropriate to the task. This is what Simon Borg-Olivier refers to as the *bandhas* (or joint complex cocontractions) in yoga, which are discussed in subsequent chapters.[23] Control of the mobility of the spine requires the ability to create stiffness in segments above and below the area of desired movement. This is very dynamic and requires spontaneous organization of a skilled mover. If this mover were to attempt to volitionally hold or stabilize the local stabilizers, the timing of that natural and spontaneous contraction would be impaired. These contractions seem to be much faster than a conscious contraction, as shown by Hodges and Richardson.[24] In this famous 1996

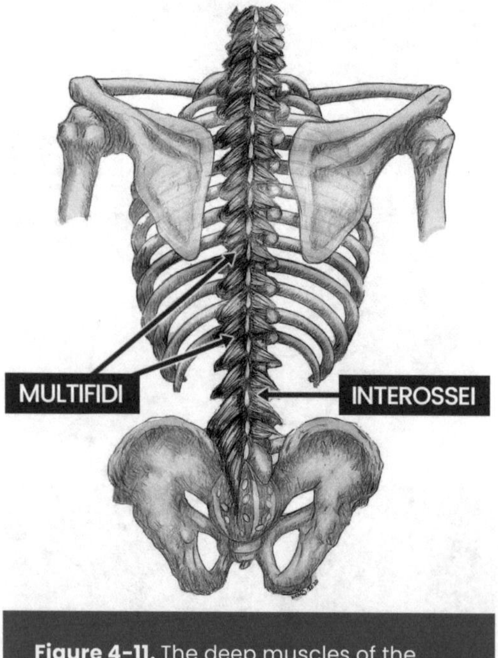

MULTIFIDI   INTEROSSEI

Figure 4-11. The deep muscles of the back.
(Illustrated by Kelly Anderson.)

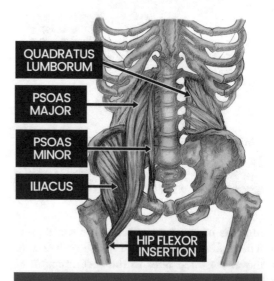

QUADRATUS LUMBORUM

PSOAS MAJOR

PSOAS MINOR

ILIACUS

HIP FLEXOR INSERTION

Figure 4-12. The psoas anterior view.
(Illustrated by Kelly Anderson.)

study by Hodges and Richardson,[24] the transverse abdominis firing was consistently 50 milliseconds faster than the intended global contraction. This suggests that the neuromuscular firing was probably a spinal cord response to the anticipated load because the amount of time it would take to be a conscious contraction in its fastest incidence would be around 300 milliseconds. It could also be part of a learned and preprogrammed firing based on an anticipation that regulates through the proprioceptive system. I expand on this concept in the Motor Control section. Let us return to the muscle anatomy of the spine. As you can imagine in the spine with 24 motion segments, smooth spine articulation in any plane would require both segmental stiffness and mobility to achieve fluidity, as observed in a beautiful golf swing. The golf club follows a sequence of rotation and derotation of the entire axial skeleton, including the upper and lower extremities. As the golf club accelerates, the golfer addresses the ball with precision. On a side note, if a golfer were to think about each joint and every muscle, it would take hours to swing the club.

I keep mentioning appropriate stiffness and anticipated load. The anticipation is based on experience. The more practice we have in a movement sequence, the more efficient the local stabilizers work to create optimal dynamic stabilization. The key word is practice.

NONCONTRACTILE STRUCTURES OF THE SPINE

In addition to the deep and superficial muscles, there are noncontractile structures, including ligaments, bones, tendons, discs, and fascia. It is important to define all the body's tissues as dynamically integrated and tension generating. In the biotensegrity model, which is discussed in greater depth in Chapter 5, it theoretically suggests the presence of the principle of self-regulation in the living tissues where the constant tension of these tissues plays the role of discontinuous compression,

and without the surrounding tension-generating muscles and tension-resisting tendons, ligaments, and fascia, bones and cartilage would do little to support our upright posture.[25,26]

The anterior longitudinal ligament is a very strong ligament that lies along the front of the spine (Figure 4-13). It prevents the lumbar spine from collapsing or shifting forward, which in humans is very important as a bipedal animal. On the backside of the lumbar curve is another ligament called the *posterior longitudinal ligament* (see Figure 4-13). Notice in Figure 4-13 that in the lumbar spine the posterior longitudinal ligament is smaller than the anterior longitudinal ligament. This again is about the efficiency of a bipedal animal with a bicurve spine. The lordotic side of the spine does not need as much ligamentous support in standing, walking, jumping, or running. It is only in the last 100 years that we have become more sedentary, increasing the demand for a stronger posterior longitudinal ligament. Unfortunately, or fortunately, our anatomy has not evolved yet for today's sedentary lifestyle. It is becoming an epidemic based on our society's choice of activities (eg, prolonged sitting).[27,28] For that reason, we are seeing an increase in lower back pathology, obesity, and other metabolic disorders.

Another important ligament is the ligamentum flavum (see Figure 4-13). The elastin inside of the tissue makes it more yellow, and it has an elastic property. Its placement is just behind the spinal canal, and it can stretch and recoil unlike the anterior and posterior longitudinal ligaments. The elasticity of the ligamentum flavum allows for noncontractile stability posteriorly to the central axis of the spinal segments and throughout their normal ranges of movement.

There are other small ligaments like the interspinous and intertransverse ligaments. These ligaments segmentally connect the transverse process and the spinous process and provide inert segmental stability at the end of range. They are also thought by some anatomists to be so thin that their primary purpose

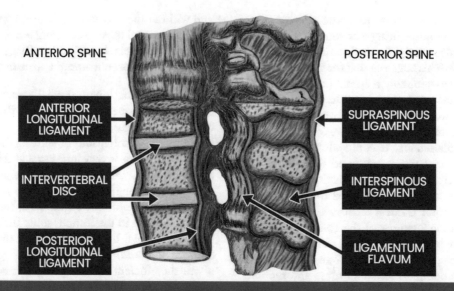

ANTERIOR SPINE

POSTERIOR SPINE

ANTERIOR
LONGITUDINAL
LIGAMENT

INTERVERTEBRAL
DISC

POSTERIOR
LONGITUDINAL
LIGAMENT

SUPRASPINOUS
LIGAMENT

INTERSPINOUS
LIGAMENT

LIGAMENTUM
FLAVUM

Figure 4-13. The ligaments of the spine.

(Illustrated by Kelly Anderson.)

might be to separate or connect the myofascial layers in the spine.[3] We do not often talk about the spinal ligaments like we do the ligaments of the knee or ankle. To help us better understand spinal ligaments, we can compare them with the ligaments of the ankle. The ankle sprain is the most common orthopedic injury; the ligaments can be deformed through overstretching, or worse, rupture, and lose their ability to provide accurate proprioceptive feedback to the nervous system through the mechanoreceptors embedded in the ligament tissue. A damaged ligament also cannot provide mechanical stability to the joint, especially at the end of range. The spinal ligaments are no different; if they have been strained severely enough, the ligament can become deformed or can rupture. According to Manohar Panjabi's triangle of stability (ie, contractile tissues, inert tissues, and motor control), when the inert or noncontractile structures are damaged, the neurologic and contractile tissues must compensate. It is like someone losing one of their senses. If someone loses their sight, the other senses increase in their sensitivity to compensate. The local and global stabilizers need to be re-educated to provide the appropriate stiffness when the inert, noncontractile stabilizing structures have been damaged.[12]

The vertebral motion segment consists of 2 vertebrae and a disc in between. The vertebral disc can be defined by 2 parts; the middle of it is a gel-like substance referred to as the *nucleus pulposus* (Figure 4-14), and the outside of the disc is the annulus or annular rings. These fibrous rings are made up of collagen. They align in multiple planes like a woven basket. This allows the disc to resist forces of movement in all planes and create stability in multiple directions (Figure 4-15A).

BIOMECHANICS AND ARTHROKINEMATICS OF THE SPINE

Before starting with the biomechanics of the spine, I would like to discuss the planes of movement—sagittal, coronal/frontal, and horizontal/transverse. I will use a few images to aid in understanding how we move in space through these planes. All flexion and extension in the body occur in the sagittal plane (Figure 4-16). Visualize your body standing upright and a pane of glass splitting your

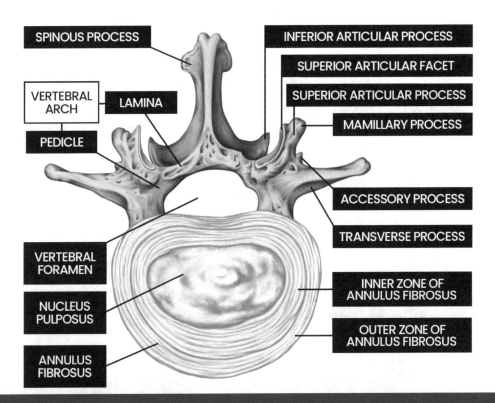

SPINOUS PROCESS

VERTEBRAL ARCH — LAMINA

PEDICLE

VERTEBRAL FORAMEN

NUCLEUS PULPOSUS

ANNULUS FIBROSUS

INFERIOR ARTICULAR PROCESS

SUPERIOR ARTICULAR FACET

SUPERIOR ARTICULAR PROCESS

MAMILLARY PROCESS

ACCESSORY PROCESS

TRANSVERSE PROCESS

INNER ZONE OF ANNULUS FIBROSUS

OUTER ZONE OF ANNULUS FIBROSUS

Figure 4-14. A disc with the nucleus pulposus.   (stihii/Shutterstock.com.)

body into a right and left side. If you move parallel to the pane of glass, you are moving in the sagittal plane. Another way of remembering the word sagittal is to associate it with the saddle of a horse. When you are sitting on the saddle of the horse, your movement is forward and backward (ie, flexion and extension). Movements in the sagittal plane include marching, swinging your arms front and back, and doing a somersault.

The next plane of movement is the coronal or frontal plane. Imagine a pane of glass separating the body into a front and a back half or anterior and posterior parts. All side-bending movement is in this plane, and all abduction/adduction of the extremities is in the coronal plane (see Figure 4-16). A cartwheel or a jumping jack takes place in the coronal plane.

The third plane of movement is the transverse or horizontal plane. Imagine the pane of glass dividing the body into an upper and lower half. The motion that is associated with the transverse plane is rotation. This includes axial rotation and rotation of the extremities. All rotation occurs in the horizontal or transverse plane (see Figure 4-16). If you look back over your shoulder, that is movement in the transverse plane.

When we describe movement or exercises in medical or professional circles, we often refer to a motion in the corresponding plane of movement. The starting position is what we refer to as the *anatomical position* (see Figure 4-16). The planes of movement are associated with the body's orientation with itself and not with gravity. We do this to improve the clarity in describing movement patterns and exercises so that we are comparing apples to apples. Exercises like a standing roll down and sit-ups

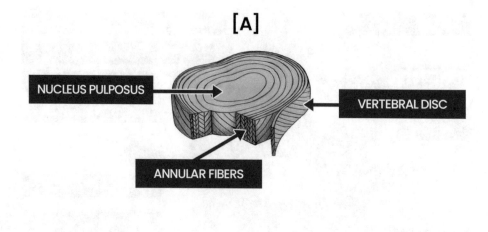

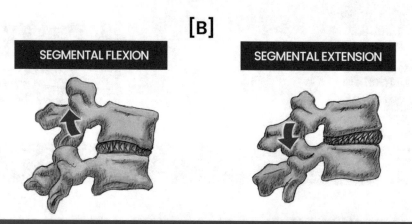

Figure 4-15. (A) Disc with annular fibers and nucleus pulposus. (B) Tripod weight-bearing between vertebral segments anteriorly through the disc and posteriorly through the facets.

(Illustrated by Kelly Anderson.)

lying down on the mat are both examples of spine flexion in the sagittal plane even though they are in different orientations to the ground.

Let us discuss the facets of the spine, which I believe are important to understand to fully embrace spine mobility. The facets of the vertebrae project posterolaterally from the pedicles and connect the vertebrae (one to another). The facet joint, also known as the *zygapophysial joint* or the *posterior tripod of the articulating segment*, is made up of the inferior articulating process of the vertebra above with the superior articulating process of the vertebra below (see Figure 4-15B). These joints are

typical synovial joints with cartilage, a synovial membrane, and fluid and are surrounded by a joint capsule.[3]

As I mentioned at the beginning of this principle, the angle of the facets determines the bias of movement found in the different sections of the spine. In each of the sections of the spine, we can find unique mechanical features that shed light on the amount and direction of spinal movement.

In the lumbar spine, the facets are vertically oriented in the sagittal plane (Figure 4-17A). In lumbar flexion, the superior vertebral

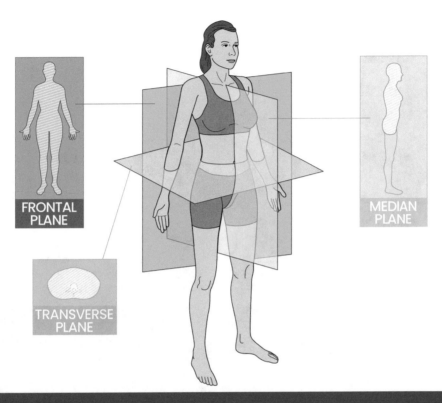

FRONTAL
PLANE

MEDIAN
PLANE

TRANSVERSE
PLANE

Figure 4-16. A diagram of the planes of movement: median/sagittal plane, transverse/
horizontal plane, and frontal/coronal plane. (Excellent Dream/Shutterstock.com.)

segment pivots over the disc as the inferior facets slide forward over the superior facets of the
vertebra below. In flexion, this movement is
limited by the tension of the facet capsule and
posterior ligaments. Extension of the vertebral
segment is usually limited by the closure of the
facet joint and approximation of the spinous
processes.[3] When the facets of the lumbar
glide bilaterally, flexion and extension occur. If
the vertebral segment glides unilaterally, there
is lateral flexion. Lateral flexion can be considered the second motion of the lumbar facets,
whereas flexion and extension in the sagittal
plane are the primary motions of the lumbar
spine. Because of the vertical nature and the
sagittal facings of the facets at 90 degrees,
rotation is the most limited (as little as 3 to 5
degrees per segment).[3]

Like the lumbar spine, the primary movements of the thoracic facet joints are flexion and
extension. Observe in Figures 4-17A through
4-17C how the facets of the thoracic spine glide
in flexion and extension. The difference occurs
with unilateral movement when the change
to a coronally oriented facet results in rotation instead of lateral flexion or side bending.
Remember the difference between the lumbar
and thoracic spine is primarily distinguished
by the orientation and angle of the facet joints.
Lastly, there is a limited amount of lateral flexion; like the lumbar facets limit rotation, the
thoracic facets limit lateral flexion and so does
the orientation of space between the ribs. If you
have ever measured side bending, you might
note that collectively there is still a substantial
amount of lateral flexion available in the thoracic spine. Even a little lateral flexion from each of
the 12 segments in the thoracic spine can add up.

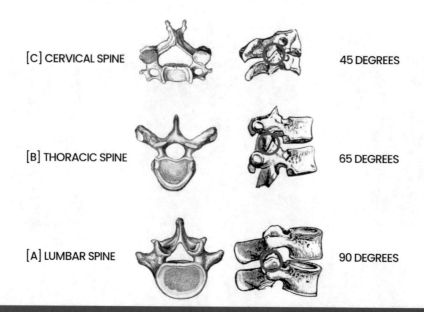

[C] CERVICAL SPINE   45 DEGREES

[B] THORACIC SPINE   65 DEGREES

[A] LUMBAR SPINE   90 DEGREES

Figure 4-17. Facets of the spine: (a) the lumbar spine, (b) the thoracic spine, and the (c) cervical spine.

The thoracic spine has several interesting movement properties. Even though we often refer to the transition joint of the thoracic-lumbar junction as T12-L1, the actual transition joint is T11-12. The facets change their orientation from a sagittal plane facet at 90 degrees to a coronal plane facet that has about a 65-degree inclination (see Figure 4-17B).[3,11] At T12, there is an interesting posterior protuberance that marks the change in orientation between sagittal-oriented facets and coronal-oriented facets (Figure 4-18). This protuberance makes T11-12 the transition joint between thoracic movement properties and lumbar movement properties. This is where in bipedal activity (ie, activities on 2 feet), lateral motion of the lumbopelvic area is converted into rotational energy in the thorax, enhancing the performance of the upper extremities.

It is important to note that there is also a difference between motion in the upper and the lower thoracic spine. In the lower thoracic spine, the primary order of movement planes from most to least movement is as follows: flexion/extension, rotation, and lateral flexion.

In the upper thoracic spine (ie, levels T1-7), there is a different order; the primary plane of movement is rotation, then flexion/extension, and then lateral flexion.[12] The upper extremity receives its power from the legs. There is a transference of force originating in the lower extremities, through the pelvis and lumbar spine, continuing up through the thoracic spine, through the scapula, and into the upper extremity. The reverse is true as well, transferring the force from the upper extremity through the scapula into the upper thorax, lower thorax, lumbar spine and pelvis, and lower extremities. Think of throwing a baseball and how the entire body is used to support the whipping action of the upper extremity. When someone throws a ball just from the upper extremity, it is not very effective, whereas someone who uses their whole body can throw with great speed and distance. If you look at the anatomy, you will notice that the scapula rests on the first 7 ribs, and the upper thorax acts as the structural support for the scapulae and upper extremities. Rotation in the upper thoracic spine gives us increased dexterity and suppleness with the use of our

THORACIC VERTEBRAE T12: LATERAL VIEW

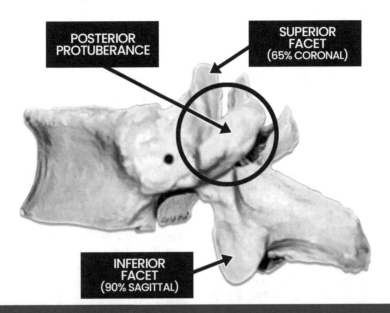

POSTERIOR PROTUBERANCE

SUPERIOR FACET (65% CORONAL)

INFERIOR FACET (90% SAGITTAL)

Figure 4-18. T12.

(sciencepics/Shutterstock.com.)

BOX 4-1: SUMMARY OF SPINE MECHANICS

Lumbar spine: The primary function is to bear weight; it has a primary motion of flexion/extension and a secondary motion of lateral flexion; the third and most limited plane of motion is rotation.

Lower thoracic spine: The primary movement is flexion and extension (like the lumbar spine) and then rotation and lateral flexion.

Upper thoracic spine: The primary movement is rotation to support the upper extremity, then flexion and extension, and finally lateral flexion.

Cervical spine: The primary function is to support and move the head. C3-7 have coronal facets that are at an approximate 45-degree orientation and account collectively for 50% of the head's movement in all 3 planes. The occiput and C1 and C2 account for the other 50% of the head's movement in all 3 planes.

This summary is provided with the assumption that the spine is in its optimal posture. For example, slouched shoulders, a kyphotic thoracic spine, and a forward head will all decrease the available movement of the head and upper and lower extremities simply by removing available movement of the capsules and ligaments of the cervical vertebrae, reducing the available range of motion and increasing the risk of end-of-range trauma or degeneration.

upper extremities in our daily lives. This is explored in greater depth when the upper extremity and lower extremity biomechanics are discussed in the principle of alignment.

The cervical facets (C3-7) have a coronal orientation of about 45 degrees and can move amply in all 3 planes (see Figure 4-17C). C1 and C2 are unique in their orientation and in how C1 articulates with the skull. C1 and C2 are like 2 plates stacked on top of each other; there is a little bone that comes up from C2 that is called the *dens* (see Figure 4-8). The biomechanics of the skull and C1 can be compared to a ball in a shallow bowl, acting more like a shallow ball-and-socket joint. The head moves in the concavity of C1 like a ball moving in a slippery bowl; it can move forward and backward and side to side.

As we better understand the biomechanics of the spine, especially the facets of the spine, it becomes easier to appreciate the ability of our spines to move in all planes. Because of the magnificent design of the axial skeleton, in particular the spine, our potential of movement combinations is quite endless, as can be observed with one of my favorite performing troupes, Cirque du Soleil.

DISC MECHANICS

Julius Wolff's law is very important as it relates to biomechanics.[29] Wolff said that our bone tissues adapt to the stresses that are applied to them. It is kind of like the adage of "use it or lose it" or "we are what we practice." There is research that shows that our connective tissue adapts to stresses applied or not applied.[30] Like all tissues, the disc tissue needs to experience a regular 3-dimensional load to have proper tissue adaptation. In many movement forms, such as Pilates, Gyrotonic Expansion System, yoga, and martial arts, the sequencing of the exercises moves and loads the spine and body tissues in all planes and orientations. Prohibiting or cautioning against moving in one plane or a combination of planes is counterintuitive to the nature of human movement. As movement practitioners,

it is necessary to explore movement through all planes, including combined planes, to facilitate functional tissue adaptation in the disc fibers, bones, tendons, and ligaments, resulting in an increased resistance to compression and tensile forces during functional activities of daily living. The key here is load modification, which is discussed in Chapter 6.

Here is where I give my multiplanar movement disclaimer. If you or your client have been living a sedentary life for years and only participate in sagittal plane movements (eg, sitting in a chair or putting on your shoes), your tissues will require a movement restoration plan to prepare the tissues to tolerate load in multiplanar movements. It may be obvious how important it is to condition all systems of the body to run a marathon and that it might take 6 to 12 months to get the body ready for a race. It is the same for any new activity we ask of our bodies. It is common that individuals, after years of sitting at a desk, jump right into playing tennis or golf. Just as one would start off slow and gradually increase their mileage preparing for a marathon, increasing tissue tolerance to the rotation of a tennis or golf swing needs the same preparation. This might take 6 months to 1 year with a graded load and graded mobility restoration plan to (re)create healthy, elastic tissues able to perform normal human function, something we refer to in Polestar as *the human's right to move*.

We very seldom move in only one plane; most movement occurs in a combination of all planes. To better understand this, we apply Harrison Fryette's laws. Fryette's laws are biomechanical laws that we often refer to in spine treatment, particularly in manual therapy. Fryette's third law states that when motion is introduced in one plane, it will modify (reduce) the available motion in the other 2 planes.[31] Let me clarify this. If flexion is introduced to a spinal motion segment (eg, bending forward) followed by rotation (eg, tying your shoes), there will be less available rotation and flexion through those segments compared with isolated flexion or rotation initiated from a neutral position.

We can observe that a successful golf swing requires rotation in the spine and the extremities. The desired rotation should be distributed through the body, beginning with the thoracic spine, especially the upper thoracic, and then a little from the lumbar spine and then the lower extremities. According to Fryette's law, if the golfer approaches the golf ball with rounded shoulders, a flat back, and a tucked pelvis, you can begin to see that the availability of rotation in the spine and hips will be greatly reduced. It is no surprise that so many golfers complain of low back, shoulder, hip, and knee pain, not to mention elbow and wrist problems. Like water, movement flows where there is the least resistance, even if it is not the safest or most ideal strategy. Axial elongation and proper alignment of the spine and extremities will increase segmental mobility, especially in the plane of rotation necessary for the swing, and hopefully improve the performance of the golfer (Figure 4-19). I always promise my golf clients that I can increase their drive by 20 yards; I just cannot promise in which direction. Now you know my secret.

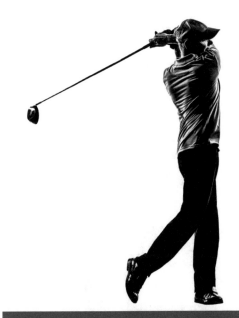

Figure 4-19. The golfer's swing.
(Frank Camhi/Shutterstock.com.)

LOWER EXTREMITY ANATOMY AND BIOMECHANICS

BONY ANATOMY OF THE LOWER EXTREMITY

Let us now move into observing the anatomy of the lower extremity (Figures 4-20A and 4-20B). The pelvis is the central distribution area of all lower extremity weight-bearing and the link to the axial skeleton. All ground reaction forces pass through the pelvis into the spine. It has a shape like a shell or a bowl that holds the weight and contents of our viscera. It connects to the spine that holds our torso, head, and upper extremities. It balances on top of the femoral head. It is quite a miracle that our body can balance on one foot against gravity. If you have ever tried to build a structure with vertical sticks and have them stand up, typically, you must bring things from the outside to hold them up or wedge them in. The biotensegrity of the myofascial system provides the proper tension and compression to balance the vertical skeleton on a single leg.

The relationship between the pelvis and the top of the femoral head becomes incredibly important with all upright postures. The femoral head is balanced almost directly under the ala of the sacrum. When beginning to stand on one leg, one only needs a minimal lateral shift to find balance. From the ball and socket, the femoral neck angles inferiorly and laterally in the coronal plane to create the most amazing myofascial force couple that allows efficient single-leg weight-bearing. The femoral shaft then angles back toward the midline to articulate with the tibia. The femoral condyles and their articulation with the tibial plateau are another amazing biomechanical design. I believe the condyles determine the arthrokinematics of the entire lower extremity. The medial condyle is larger than the lateral condyle. The condyles balance on top of the tibia, the

[A] LATERAL VIEW

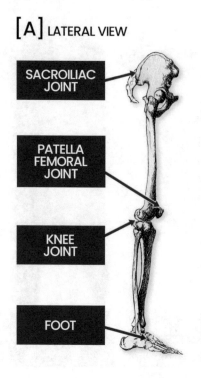

SACROILIAC JOINT

PATELLA FEMORAL JOINT

KNEE JOINT

FOOT

[B] ANTERIOR VIEW

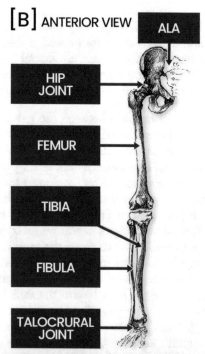

ALA

HIP JOINT

FEMUR

TIBIA

FIBULA

TALOCRURAL JOINT

Figure 4-20. The lower extremity skeleton. (A) The lateral view and (B) the anterior view.

main weight-bearing bone in the lower leg. The tibia descends from the knee and with the fibula articulates with the ankle or the talus. The relationship between the distal tibia and fibula makes up the talocrural joint with the talus of the foot. The dome of the talus is slightly wider anteriorly and is designed to create an inert tension in dorsiflexion and initial supination of the forefoot when toeing off in gait.

The foot anatomy can be a book in and of itself. I love to look at the foot and break it down by its function. Initially, the foot can be divided into 2 parts. The lateral foot (Figure 4-21) consists of the calcaneus (heel), which articulates with the cuboid; the cuboid articulates with the 4th and 5th metatarsals and their phalanges (toes). The primary movements associated with the lateral foot are eversion and inversion. The medial foot consists of the talus, which articulates with the navicular, and the navicular bone articulates with the cuneiform bones and then the 1st, 2nd, and 3rd metatarsals, which articulate with the phalanges (see Figure 4-21). The primary movements of the medial portion of the foot are pronation and supination.

MUSCLES OF THE LOWER EXTREMITY

The myofascial anatomy of the superior aspect of the lower extremity can be divided into 3 subdivisions: anterior, medial, and posterior. The anterior compartment consists of the vastus lateralis, vastus intermedius, vastus medialis, rectus femoris, and sartorius muscles (Figures 4-22 and 4-23). The medial compartment consists of the adductors, including the adductor magnus (see Figures 4-22 and 4-23). The posterior compartment of the thigh consists of the hamstrings, 4 muscles that help control hip extension and knee flexion (ie, the semitendinosus, semimembranosus, short and long head of the biceps femoris, and adductor magnus; see Figures 4-22A and 4-22B). Note the relationship of the fascia and the connective tissue around each of the muscles in Figure 4-23A.

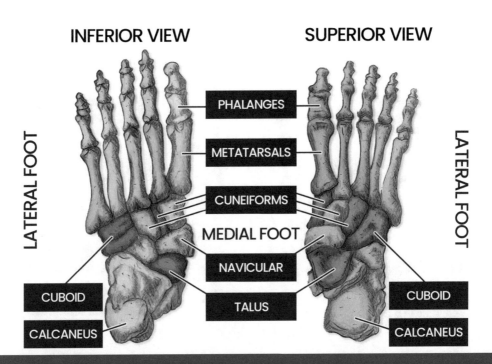

INFERIOR VIEW   SUPERIOR VIEW

LATERAL FOOT

PHALANGES

METATARSALS

CUNEIFORMS

MEDIAL FOOT

NAVICULAR

CUBOID

TALUS

CUBOID

CALCANEUS

CALCANEUS

LATERAL FOOT

Figure 4-21. A view of the foot.   (Illustrated by Kelly Anderson.)

If you were to stand up right now and feel your leg muscles, you would notice that they are not that stiff. If you shifted your weight onto one leg and lifted the other leg, you would notice that the tone in the muscle increases. Every muscle fiber is enveloped by fascia. The fascia latae surrounds the whole thigh and is reinforced laterally by the iliotibial band. These muscles, and all muscles, work in harmony to create enough stiffness to complete a task, such as standing on one leg. If we tried to tell the muscles how much to contract, we would probably be wrong. From the earlier experience of standing on one leg, you noticed the thigh became a little bit stiffer to balance on top of the single leg. When you returned to 2 legs, they relaxed again. It is very dynamic. When was the last time you thought about walking, running, or putting something up on a high shelf? I bet you did not have the following conversation with your body: "As I step forward, I need to contract my quads to straighten my knee, ooh, and my outer hip muscles to stay upright. And here come the hamstrings to help me bend my

knee" and so on. You would never get anywhere if that were the case. Typically, walking is done by gravity and momentum. We mostly use our muscles to decelerate our motion in gait so that we do not fall. The more we incline our vertical axis, the more gravity moves us toward the gait pattern we know as running. The more vertical our axis, the more likely we are to walk. I often refer to walking and running as *controlled falling*—the faster we locomote, the more we rely on the elasticity of the myofascial tissues.

The muscle groups of the lower leg are also compartmentalized (see Figure 4-23B). The muscle groups in the anterior compartment consist of the tibialis anterior and the extensors of the foot in the toes. The lateral leg muscles consist of the peroneus brevis and longus. The posterior deep muscles consist of the long flexors of the foot and ankle, the soleus, and then superficially the gastrocnemius (see Figure 4-23B). The lower leg muscles work synergistically to provide stiffness, acceleration, deceleration, and proprioception of where the

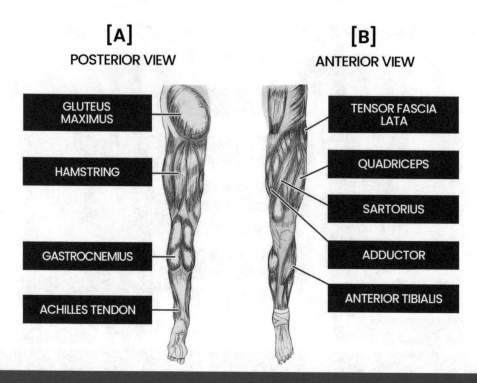

[A]
POSTERIOR VIEW

GLUTEUS MAXIMUS

HAMSTRING

GASTROCNEMIUS

ACHILLES TENDON

[B]
ANTERIOR VIEW

TENSOR FASCIA LATA

QUADRICEPS

SARTORIUS

ADDUCTOR

ANTERIOR TIBIALIS

Figure 4-22. Muscles of the lower extremity. (A) The posterior view and (B) the anterior view of the thigh.
(Illustrated by Kelly Anderson.)

body is in space and its relationship to the ground. Like the thigh, the leg is surrounded by fascia from the muscle fascicle to the fascia that surrounds the entire leg (see Figure 4-23B). Many of the muscles cross multiple joints; the muscle spindle fibers and Golgi organs in the tendons provide dynamic proprioception of where the body is in space. The fascia is also filled with Golgi organs, which have the primary purpose of providing antigravity awareness. This becomes more obvious when someone has experienced an injury to the lower extremity and a temporary loss of their feedback mechanisms through the fascia, tendons, and muscle spindle fibers. They often will make statements such as "I don't know whose leg this is" or "Wow, I can hardly stand on one leg." After rehabilitation, the feedback mechanisms are restored, and they forgot that they had that problem.

A very beautiful concept is that our muscles work efficiently to try to maintain our uprightness and the efficiency of our movement. Isolated training of the quadriceps (eg, to improve stair-climbing) will never be as effective as climbing stairs. Function requires coordination of all the muscles in the area, not one working by itself.

Less desirable movement impairments can be caused by our sedentary lifestyle and include poor ankle dorsiflexion, poor lateral hip stability, poor hip extension in standing, and poor alignment of the torso and pelvis. The loss of mobility, alignment, and load tolerance has greatly diminished our ability to efficiently participate in normal human activities that depend greatly on proper dynamic alignment of the bones, correct tensile forces from the connective tissues, and repetition of the desired activity until it becomes spontaneous and natural.

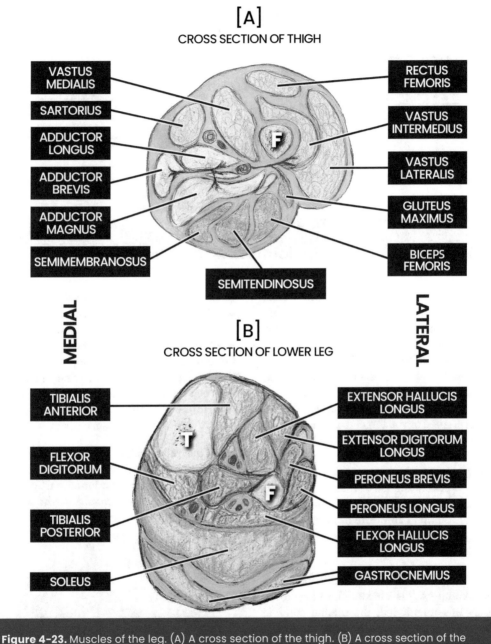

[A]
CROSS SECTION OF THIGH

VASTUS MEDIALIS

SARTORIUS

ADDUCTOR LONGUS

ADDUCTOR BREVIS

ADDUCTOR MAGNUS

SEMIMEMBRANOSUS

SEMITENDINOSUS

RECTUS FEMORIS

VASTUS INTERMEDIUS

VASTUS LATERALIS

GLUTEUS MAXIMUS

BICEPS FEMORIS

F

MEDIAL

LATERAL

[B]
CROSS SECTION OF LOWER LEG

TIBIALIS ANTERIOR

FLEXOR DIGITORUM

TIBIALIS POSTERIOR

SOLEUS

EXTENSOR HALLUCIS LONGUS

EXTENSOR DIGITORUM LONGUS

PERONEUS BREVIS

PERONEUS LONGUS

FLEXOR HALLUCIS LONGUS

GASTROCNEMIUS

T

F

Figure 4-23. Muscles of the leg. (A) A cross section of the thigh. (B) A cross section of the lower leg. (Illustrated by Kelly Anderson.)

BIOMECHANICS OF THE LOWER EXTREMITY

Let us start with the hip. The hip itself is a ball-and-socket joint (Figure 4-24). It is a deep socket joint with very strong ligaments. The ligaments and capsule around it are very thick and strong with little elasticity. They hold the head of the femur in place to maintain congruence between the joint surfaces. This optimizes weight distribution and the absorption of forces in the joint. The term *congruence* is

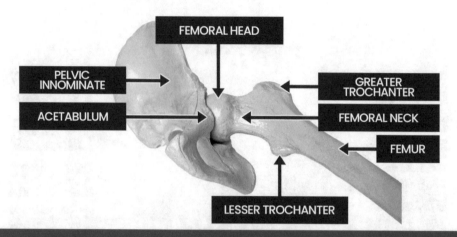

Figure 4-24. The hip joint.

used to define the optimal contact between the 2 articulating surfaces of the joint. A joint that has poor congruence will experience abnormal tissue load, which can result in degeneration, or if the surfaces of the joint do not have weight-bearing, they can also suffer degeneration because of poor joint nutrition. It is like the tires on your car wearing out because the axles were not aligned or you forgot to rotate the tires. There is uneven wear and tear. The labrum of the hip deepens the socket and increases the stability while providing absorption of forces. If the joint is poorly aligned or there is poor neuromuscular organization around the hip, the torque of rotation can create abnormal forces that can damage the articulating cartilage or the labrum (Figure 4-25).

The knee joint may not seem like it, but it is quite complex. It is a bicondylar hinge joint, and, as was mentioned, the medial condyle is larger than the lateral condyle, creating a unique spiral between the femur and tibia when the knee bends and straightens (Figures 4-26A and 4-26B). This is important to understand. It is like a hand truck that has 2 wheels, and one is much bigger than the other one. When the wheels spin forward or backward, it will create a spiral. It is not a physiological rotation like internal/external rotation but rather an accessory motion. When the knee bends, the medial condyle spirals laterally,

resulting in a lateral spiral of the femur. This relationship reciprocally causes a medial spiral of the tibia and can be compared to the lid on a jar. To tighten or loosen the lid requires the lid and the jar to move in opposite directions (Figures 4-27A and 4-27B). The spiral force between the long bones increases the stability and stiffness of the joint and maintains the congruence of the joint surfaces.

This relationship of one condyle being bigger than the other creates an accessory joint movement as mentioned earlier and is known as the *arthrokinematics* or the *science of*

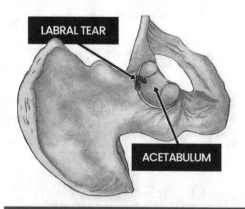

Figure 4-25. A labral tear.

(Illustrated by Kelly Anderson.)

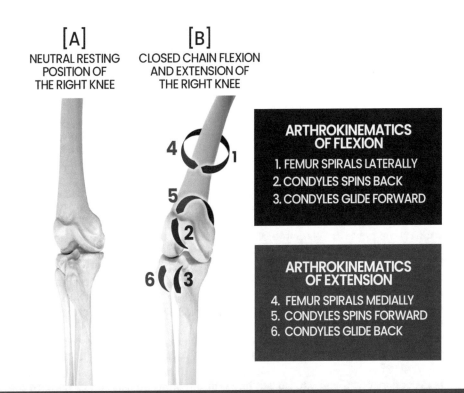

[A]
NEUTRAL RESTING
POSITION OF
THE RIGHT KNEE

[B]
CLOSED CHAIN FLEXION
AND EXTENSION OF
THE RIGHT KNEE

ARTHROKINEMATICS OF FLEXION
1. FEMUR SPIRALS LATERALLY
2. CONDYLES SPINS BACK
3. CONDYLES GLIDE FORWARD

ARTHROKINEMATICS OF EXTENSION
4. FEMUR SPIRALS MEDIALLY
5. CONDYLES SPINS FORWARD
6. CONDYLES GLIDE BACK

Figure 4-26. Right knee joint arthrokinematics. (A) The neutral resting position. (B) Closed chain flexion and extension.

accessory joint movement. Accessory motions are different from physiological movements (eg, flexion, extension, abduction, rotation, and pronation). Accessory motions happen inside the joint to allow physiological movement and are often identified as spin, roll, glide, and spiral. One of the accessory motions of the knee joint is a spiral. This is an amazing coupling of accessory movements that, when dynamically aligned, optimize load absorption through the myofascial system.[30,32-34] The spiral of the knee creates a certain amount of tension in the fascia in multiple planes. When we are standing and moving, the tension through the fascia has a beautiful balancing relationship between the pelvis and the upper body, which allows us to be upright. I remind you that we are the only upright animal that has a bicurve spine. Even our cousins, the primates, have a C-curve spine (Figure 4-28), which does not allow them to stand upright, at least not efficiently.

When the arthrokinematics of the lower extremity joints function correctly, there is alignment and improved power. The menisci and the ligaments are protected through the correct dynamic alignment. However, if both the femur and the tibia spiral internally, it will result in a valgus stress, putting the ligaments and the menisci at risk of degeneration and injury. Another name in the dance and movement world for arthrokinematics is *bone rhythms.*[35]

The ankle, also known as the *talocrural joint*, is made up of the malleoli of the tibia and fibula with the talus (Figure 4-29). It is also a complex joint. The dome of the talus looks a bit like a saddle for a horse (Figure 4-30). The anterior aspect of the dome is wider than the posterior aspect. When the inferior articulating surfaces of the tibia and fibula articulate with the dome of the talus into dorsiflexion,

BOX 4-2: BONE RHYTHMS IN THE LOWER EXTREMITY EXERCISE

Stand with your feet shoulder-width apart and your legs slightly turned out. The key objective is to allow the joints to follow their normal arthrokinematics/bone rhythms. Just like the jar and lid, the bones on each side of the joint will need to spiral in opposite directions. Use the following images to compare natural vs unnatural imagery to facilitate a healthy squat strategy.

1. Imagine the pelvis spiraling medially (pubic bones narrowing/sit bones widening), the femurs spiraling laterally, and the tibias spiraling medially as you squat. Reverse the spirals on the return to standing.

2. Imagine the pelvis spiraling laterally (pubic bones widening/sit bones narrowing), the femurs spiraling medially, and the tibias spiraling laterally as you squat. Reverse the spirals on the return to standing.

3. Imagine the pelvis, femur, and tibial spiraling laterally as you squat, and reverse the spiraling on the return to standing.

4. Imagine the pelvis, femur, and tibial spiraling medially as you squat, and reverse the spiraling on the return to standing.

Which of the 4 imagery techniques felt most natural when squatting? What did you notice about the depth of the squat, the muscle tone, and joint stressors with each of the 4 strategies?

Modification: If you feel you do not have ample ankle dorsiflexion to perform the squat, place a 2- to 3-inch lift under the heels and repeat the squatting activities.

[A]
OPENING JAR

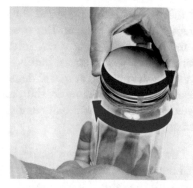

EQUAL AND OPPOSITE
FORCES TO OPEN LID

[B]
CLOSING JAR

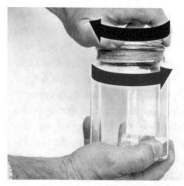

EQUAL AND OPPOSITE
FORCES TO CLOSE LID

Figure 4-27. (A) Opening the jar: Equal and opposite forces are needed to open the lid. (B) Closing the jar: Equal and opposite forces are needed to close the lid.

COMPARED ANATOMY BETWEEN HUMAN AND PRIMATE

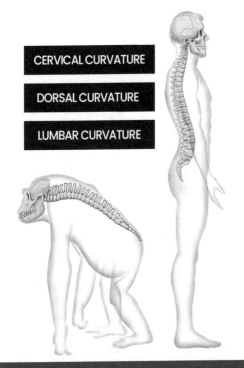

CERVICAL CURVATURE

DORSAL CURVATURE

LUMBAR CURVATURE

Figure 4-28. A comparison of the primate to the human.

(Amadeu Blasco/Shutterstock.com.)

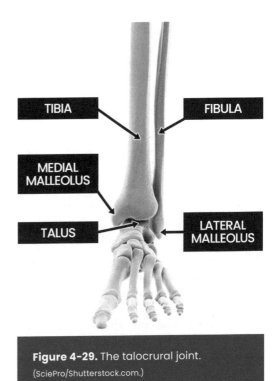

TIBIA

FIBULA

MEDIAL MALLEOLUS

TALUS

LATERAL MALLEOLUS

Figure 4-29. The talocrural joint.

(SciePro/Shutterstock.com.)

the wide anterior dome stiffens the ligaments of the talocrural joint, creating a lever that facilitates propulsion in the toe-off phase of gait.

These ligamentous structures and arthrokinematics have everything to do with natural walking, running, and jumping. When we observe prolonged pronation of the foot or other abnormal alignment patterns, it is essential to look up the kinetic chain and see what is happening in the knee and the hip. Is everything spiraling medially (ie, where the femur spirals medially, the tibia spirals medially, and all the weight collapses into a pronation of the medial foot)? Do we treat the foot or the hip? It is often the case that when clients come in with a diagnosis of excessive pronation, the first treatment is to put them into

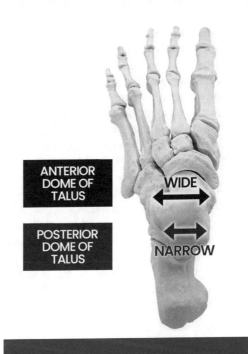

ANTERIOR DOME OF TALUS

WIDE

POSTERIOR DOME OF TALUS

NARROW

Figure 4-30. The dome of the talus.

orthotics or prepare a lift for their shoes. Instead, we should be restoring normal bone rhythms of the lower extremity and probably strengthening the hip rotators and extensors in the deceleration or loading phases of movement.

UPPER EXTREMITY ANATOMY AND BIOMECHANICS

How well the upper quadrant, including the head and neck, is organized is a powerful indicator of efficient movement. We can often look at the face or the shoulders and know if the mover is a novice or seasoned. When trained in assessment, we can also evaluate the spatial organization of the shoulder girdle in relationship to the thoracic cage, cervical spine, and head.

Pilates, yoga, gymnastics, and most martial arts all demand a lot of weight-bearing in the upper extremity. If we do not organize our upper extremities (or any part of our body) correctly, we often hang on the noncontractile tissues without neuromuscular support, which can create unnecessary stress. In upper extremity weight-bearing, this type of stress can manifest as hyperextended elbows and wrists. We can stretch out those ligaments and create hyper- or hypomobility and instability in the wrist, elbow, or shoulders. This could explain why many people who start to participate in martial arts, Pilates, or yoga will initially complain of wrist weakness and wrist pain. It is a different take on the phrase "use it or lose it." If we do not properly train and use the neuromuscular support, our joints will rely on the ligaments for support, which is inefficient and can cause wear and tear on the inert structures.

BONY ANATOMY OF THE UPPER EXTREMITY

The upper extremity anatomy begins with the spine and, some could make the claim, the pelvis. In the world of fascial science, we would of course state that these kinetic and fascial chains connect all the limbs in all planes and orientations of the body (Figure 4-31). For practical sake, let us begin with the scapula and its relationship with the head, neck, and thorax. The scapulothoracic joint is not a true joint. The scapula sits against or floats over the rib cage. It does not have a capsule, articulating cartilage, ligaments, or synovial fluid. However, it acts and functions like a joint. You can think of the scapula as tethered in all directions by myofascial tissues to maintain congruence with the rib cage and distribute forces from and through the upper extremity. The bony anatomy of the scapula is very interesting and is often described as a blade or plate in layperson's terms (shoulder blade in English and omoplato in Spanish). The curved, platelike nature of the bone is ideal for providing 2 key factors for shoulder stability. First, it can provide the proper alignment of a very dexterous limb through its range of motion and maintain congruence with the humeral head. Second, it can distribute significant force into and from the trunk in relationship to the upper extremity. I have often been so impressed by yogis, circus performers, and parkour performers and their ability to balance their entire body weight on one hand. I always observe how the myofascial tethering of the scapula to the rib cage allows for that balance and control, not to mention the alignment and congruence of the glenohumeral joint and the other long bones of the upper extremity.

The shape of the scapula bears a resemblance to the continent of South America. To best understand the organization of the scapula, we must know our bony landmarks. We can start with the medial and lateral borders of the scapula descending into the inferior angle. The spine of the scapula arises from the medial border and crosses the entire scapula

EXAMPLES OF MYOFASCIAL CONNECTIONS IN MULTIPLE PLANES

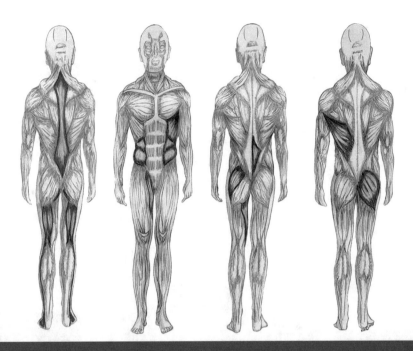

Figure 4-31. Myofascial slings. (Illustrated by Kelly Anderson.)

in a lateral superior direction, which results in the acromion process. The acromion articulates with the distal clavicle. Interestingly, the clavicle is the only true joint connection of the upper extremity to the thorax through its connection to the sternum. The lateral border of the scapula rises and develops into the glenoid fossa, which articulates with the head of the humerus. From the anterior view of the scapula, you will notice another protuberance called the *coracoid process* where the chest and arm muscles attach (Figures 4-32A and 4-32B).

The clavicle is another important bone as it relates to upper extremity mobility. The clavicle is an elongated S-shaped bone that articulates with the sternum and the acromion process of the scapula. It is the only true joint between the shoulder girdle and the thorax. The clavicle and the scapula are designed to move in a way that they maintain congruence

of the glenohumeral joint. Figure 4-33 shows the clavicle and its relationship to the spine of the scapula and how they point like a "V" to the head of the humerus. The direction of the "V" can be used for assessing shoulder girdle alignment and help determine whether there will be undue stresses in the glenohumeral joint because of poor congruence/alignment of the scapula-clavicle complex. If the shoulders are rounded, the congruence between the humerus and the glenoid fossa will be lost, and you will see the "V" pointing around to the front. If the individual overcorrects their posture (eg, a military stance pulling the shoulders back), it will result in the same thing, and you will see the "V" pointing around to the back. Ideally, we would like the "V" to point as much to the sides as possible. Remember it takes time for this area to change, both in awareness and soft tissue, so be gentle if you try to correct someone's alignment. It is a nice

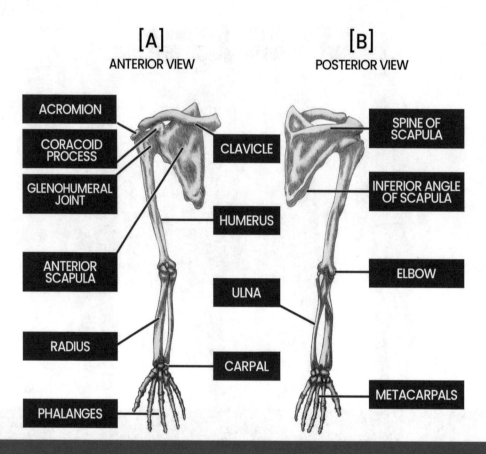

[A]
ANTERIOR VIEW

[B]
POSTERIOR VIEW

ACROMION

CORACOID PROCESS

GLENOHUMERAL JOINT

CLAVICLE

SPINE OF SCAPULA

INFERIOR ANGLE OF SCAPULA

ANTERIOR SCAPULA

HUMERUS

ELBOW

ULNA

RADIUS

CARPAL

METACARPALS

PHALANGES

Figure 4-32. Bony anatomy of the upper extremity. (A) The anterior view. (B) The posterior view.   (Illustrated by Kelly Anderson.)

little assessment trick to look at these bony alignments to know if the glenohumeral joint is at risk of strain or potential injury.

Let us continue down the chain by looking at the humerus and its anatomical features (see Figure 4-32). The head of the humerus is very big in comparison to the glenoid fossa. There are 2 protuberances around the humeral head (ie, the greater and lesser tubercle) where the rotator cuff muscles attach (Figure 4-34). The glenohumeral joint is a ball-and-socket joint providing 6 degrees of freedom like the hip. The ligamentous and capsular properties of the upper extremity are less restrictive than those found in the hip, again differentiating the agile function of the upper extremity compared with the

weight-bearing properties of the lumbopelvic region and the lower extremity. The distal end of the humerus articulates with 2 bones, the ulna and the radius. The unique fossa and protuberances create the uniplanar elbow (ie, the humeroulnar joint). The elbow only articulates in the sagittal plane because of the nature of the trochlea of the humerus and the deep trochlear notch and coronoid process of the ulna. The radius's relationship with the humerus is quite different than the ulna. Notice the convex surface of the capitulum of the humerus and the round and shallow fossa of the radial head. This allows for pronation and supination of the forearm. The radial head also articulates with the lateral aspect of the ulna in the radial notch, which contributes to pronation and supination of the forearm.

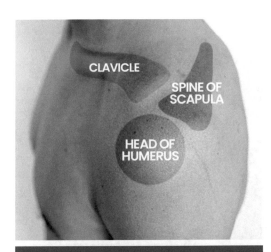

Figure 4-33. A superior view of the shoulder girdle and congruency.

(Illustrated by Kelly Anderson.)

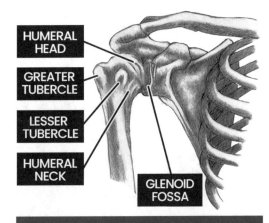

Figure 4-34. Shoulder and bony landmarks of the glenohumeral joint.

(Illustrated by Kelly Anderson.)

The distal ulna and radius articulate with the proximal row of carpal bones, with most of the bony articulation occurring with the distal radius. The distal ulna articulates indirectly through a disc with the medial proximal row of carpal bones (see Figure 4-32). The distal row of the carpal bones articulates with the 5 metacarpal bones. The most lateral of the distal row, the trapezium, articulates with the first ray or thumb and has a U-joint articulation like that of the sternoclavicular joint, which allows for opposition in the human hand. The metacarpal bones articulate with the proximal phalanges and the middle and distal phalanges to make up the fingers and thumb. Note that the thumb does not have a middle phalange, only distal (see Figure 4-32). The upper extremity anatomy provides us the ability to participate in activities that require fine motor dexterity for eating, working, sensing, and playing. The uniqueness of the upper extremity anatomy also allows for closed-chain activities (eg, planks), hanging exercises (eg, pull-ups, rock climbing), and open-chain movements (eg, throwing a ball, swinging a golf club).

MUSCULAR ANATOMY OF THE UPPER EXTREMITY

Within the shoulder girdle, we can find 3 groups of muscles. Group 1 muscles connect the scapula or clavicle to the head, neck, and trunk; group 2 muscles connect the scapula to the humerus; and group 3 muscles connect the thorax to the humerus.

Let us look at the posterior muscles in group 1 from superficial to deep (Figure 4-35). The trapezius muscle connects from the base of the head and the nuchal ligament to the spine of the scapula and all spinous processes from C2-T12. Most people think of the trapezius or "traps" as the muscle across the top of the shoulders, so it is interesting to notice how large the muscle is and how it connects all the way to the bottom of the thoracic spine. The next layer is made up of the rhomboid minor and major muscles connecting the spinous process of C7-T5 and the medial border of the scapula from the medial angle down to the inferior angle. The levator scapulae muscle originates from the transverse processes of the first 4 cervical vertebrae and inserts on the medial border of the scapula.

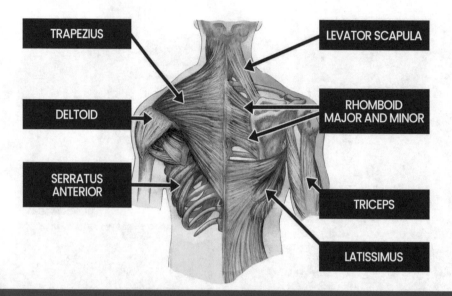

Figure 4-35. The posterior shoulder girdle muscles.   (Illustrated by Kelly Anderson.)

The anterior muscles in group 1 (Figure 4-36) include the sternocleidomastoid muscle, which originates from the manubrium and the clavicle and inserts on the mastoid process of the temporal bone of the skull, and the pectoralis minor, which connects the anterior portion of ribs 3 to 5 to the coracoid process of the scapula.

Group 2 (Figures 4-37A and 4-37B) is the grouping of muscles we often refer to as the *rotator cuff muscles*, which include the infraspinatus, supraspinatus, teres minor, and subscapularis. In addition, this group includes the deltoids, teres major, and the long head of the biceps and triceps.

Group 3 is made up of the muscles connecting the trunk to the humerus. Posteriorly, the latissimus dorsi muscle connects the humerus to the thoracolumbar fascia (Figure 4-38). Anteriorly, the pectoralis major connects the humerus to the anterior rib cage and the sternum (see Figure 4-36). Interestingly, these 2 muscles make up a major portion of the diagonal fascial slings.[30,33,34,36]

Muscles that affect the elbow and wrist are numerous, and I like to categorize them by their function as follows: elbow flexors and extensors; forearm pronators; supinators and wrist flexors; extensors, adductors, and abductors; and digit flexors, extensors, abductors, and adductors (Figures 4-39A and 4-39B). We often refer to the deep intrinsic muscles of the hand and foot in comparison to the superficial and long multijoint muscles of the hand and foot (Figures 4-40A and 4-40B). Remember that the deep muscles in the body help to support the bones and more largely the limbs or body, and the superficial muscles are mostly used to move us or to slow us down.

BIOMECHANICS OF THE UPPER EXTREMITY

The upper extremity has some unique biomechanical features that become especially important for those of us teaching closed-chain activities and sporting activities that involve the upper extremity. It is important that we first understand the primary joints of

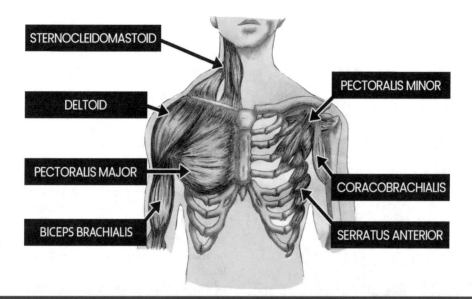

Figure 4-36. The anterior shoulder girdle muscles. (Illustrated by Kelly Anderson.)

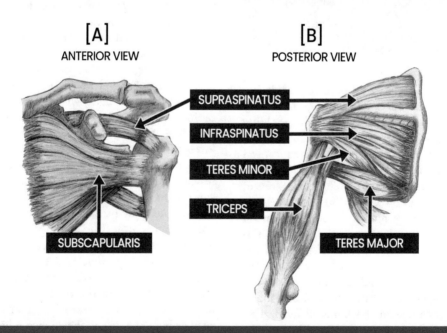

Figure 4-37. The rotator cuff muscles. (A) The anterior view. (B) The posterior view. (Illustrated by Kelly Anderson.)

LATISSIMUS DORSI MUSCLE

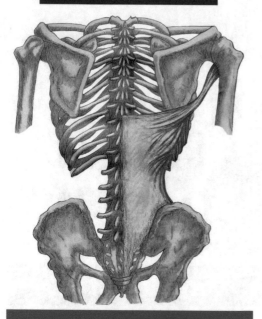

Figure 4–38. The latissimus dorsi.
(Illustrated by Kelly Anderson.)

the upper extremity. As I defined earlier, the scapulothoracic joint, or pseudo-joint, is very important to provide the balance of mobility and control for the upper extremity's mobility. The scapula must rotate on its central axis, known as *upward and downward rotations* (Figures 4-41A and 4-41B). The movement of the scapula and the clavicle makes it possible to maintain congruence of the glenohumeral joint, especially when working overhead. The scapula will rotate up and slide down the thoracic wall when the action requires the humerus to be overhead. This movement positions the glenoid fossa to dynamically maintain alignment with the humeral head. This motion of the scapula is dependent on the mobility of the thoracic spine and rib cage. If the spine cannot extend, then the scapula struggles to spiral upward and depress to optimize the relationship with the humeral head. To achieve the overhead activity, one might

force the range of motion, creating unwanted stress on the joints distal to the trunk (eg, subluxation of the glenohumeral joint or strain on the elbow, forearm, and wrist).

The elbow, forearm, and wrist create another unique biomechanical property that provides dexterity of the upper extremity. Although the elbow joint is a pure hinge joint resulting in flexion and extension, the radio-ulnar joint has unique properties at the elbow and the wrist. The radial head spins inside its ligament against the ulna, allowing the pronation and supination of the forearm. Pronation and supination are also dependent on the relationship found in the distal ulnar-radial joint. I find it interesting that the kinetic chain of bones and joints in the upper extremity, although similar to the lower extremity, are different. The humerus and ulna are a true hinge joint; yet, the distal ulna does not have a broad surface area that articulates with the proximal carpal bones through the articular disc at the medial-most part of the proximal row of carpal bones. The proximal radius does have weight-bearing properties when the arm is fully extended where the capitulum of the humerus articulates with the head of the radius like a shallow ball-and-socket joint. How is that relevant? If we compare it to the lower extremity, the tibia is the weight-bearing bone from the femur to the talus, and the fibula is not. I must assume the primary reason for the forearm mechanics always comes back to dexterity of the upper extremity, and more importantly, the hand. When we do decide to bear weight on the upper extremity, we must remember that congruence becomes even more important. We need to understand and visualize where the actual weight-bearing is taking place and avoid compensations, such as hyperextending the elbows, which can cause unwanted shear force through the joints of the upper extremity. Proper alignment and cocontractions around the joints are necessary for power, efficiency, and comfort and must be practiced, just like preparing for the marathon.

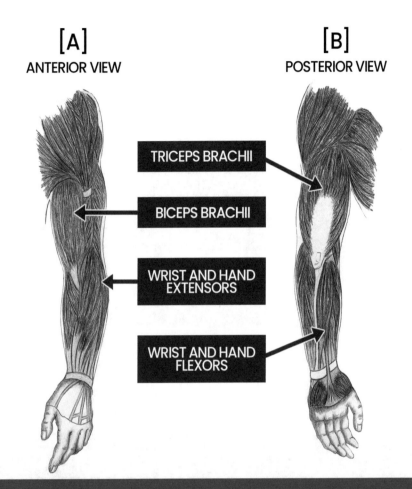

[A]
ANTERIOR VIEW

[B]
POSTERIOR VIEW

TRICEPS BRACHII

BICEPS BRACHII

WRIST AND HAND EXTENSORS

WRIST AND HAND FLEXORS

Figure 4-39. The upper extremity superficial muscles. (A) The anterior view. (B) The posterior view.   (Illustrated by Kelly Anderson.)

APPLICATION
MOTOR CONTROL

Motor control has become an incredibly popular topic, particularly in preventing and treating musculoskeletal pathologies. Healthy musculoskeletal movement occurs when neuromuscular control is smooth, efficient, and subconscious. For example, in the spine, the average human has a strategy of moving from very few spinal segments, as few as 3 to 5, when we have 24 available. The strategy of isolated mobility in a few segments in the spine increases the load on those same structures, as well as other structures in the body, and can increase the risk of injury. Increasing segmental movement by as little as 3 to 4 more segments allows for a significant distribution of force through the spine and can greatly reduce overloading the tissues that are commonly at risk of tissue failure, such as L5-S1 disc degeneration or C5-6 stenosis.

In 1996, I was part of a pilot study with the physical therapy department at Mount St. Mary's University in Southern California. We investigated segmental spine flexion from T2 to the sacrum. We recruited 20 students

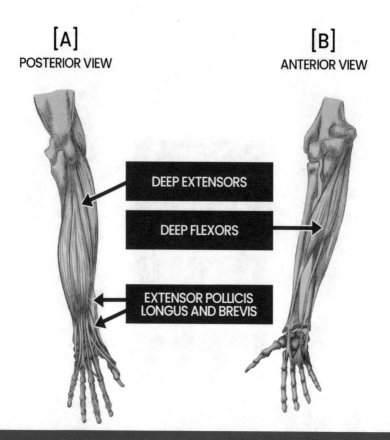

[A]
POSTERIOR VIEW

[B]
ANTERIOR VIEW

DEEP EXTENSORS

DEEP FLEXORS

EXTENSOR POLLICIS
LONGUS AND BREVIS

Figure 4-40. The upper extremity deep muscles. (A) The posterior view. (B) The anterior view. (Illustrated by Kelly Anderson.)

from the physical therapy program who had never had a complaint of back pain and had never experienced Pilates. We asked them to flex their spine (ie, forward bend) multiple times in standing; we measured the segmental displacement between each spinous process with a 3-dimensional goniometer (Metrecom Skeletal Analysis System). We also measured the total distance from their hands to the floor. The initial results showed that (1) most of the movement came from L5-S1 and L4-5, (2) there was almost no movement in the upper lumbar, and (3) there was no movement that we could measure in the thoracic spine. We then randomly assigned the 20 students to 2 different groups. One group rested for 45 minutes, came back, and tested again with the same outcomes as the initial measurement. The second group performed 45 minutes of

Pilates on the reformer. After their session, they returned to be remeasured. Three interesting findings were noted.

First, the total range of motion in flexion significantly increased after participating in a 45-minute reformer session. You might be thinking that makes sense if you did exercises that facilitated spine mobility and hamstring lengthening. An increase in their range of motion makes sense. I agree!

The second finding was that segmental movement of the upper lumbar and thoracic spine was significantly greater compared with the pre-Pilates measurement. Again, we could assume that spine articulation exercises in Pilates could increase segmental mobility of the spine.

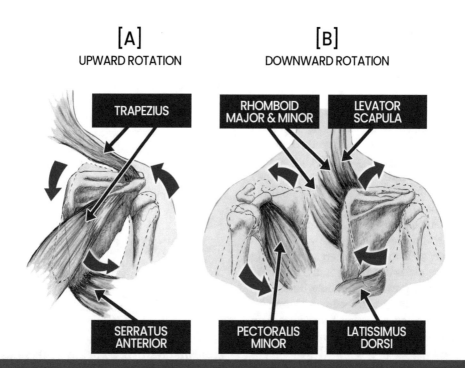

[A]
UPWARD ROTATION

[B]
DOWNWARD ROTATION

TRAPEZIUS

RHOMBOID MAJOR & MINOR

LEVATOR SCAPULA

SERRATUS ANTERIOR

PECTORALIS MINOR

LATISSIMUS DORSI

Figure 4-41. Rotation of the scapula. (A) Upward rotation. (B) Downward rotation. (Illustrated by Kelly Anderson.)

The third and most important finding was that movement at L4-5 and L5-S1 decreased by almost 50%. This is very important. We were able to facilitate a change in the participants' movement strategies after just 45 minutes of Pilates. We changed their strategy from moving primarily at the L4-5 and L5-S1 segments to having a greater range of motion overall and decreasing movement at the L4-5 and L5-S1 segments. This study is what influenced the phrase "the distribution of movement equals the distribution of force."

You can see why people with back injuries who do Pilates find that after a couple of months of faithfully performing their exercises, they now have a new movement strategy that is pain-free. They believe their back problem, disc problem, or stenosis has disappeared. It probably did not disappear, and their magnetic resonance imaging findings would likely look the same, but their strategy changed. When we look at the acquisition of new movement, we are talking about increasing access to spinal movement, which improves the distribution of the force. This might also explain why so many people notice immediate improvement with their back problems after doing Pilates or Gyrotonic Expansion System. When the teacher focuses on the mobility of joints away from the site of injury, the result is less force passing through the painful or injured segments. Changing their strategy during daily activities by adding just 2 or 3 more movement segments can drastically change their perception of well-being and pain. This makes it possible to expand their options to participate more fully in life. They often can do more than they expected, creating a paradigm shift and change in self-efficacy.

PSYCHOSOCIAL

These small successes in movement can often result in large paradigm shifts in self-efficacy and increased competence.[37,38] A return of simple activities, such as bending down to put on your shoes, getting a bar of soap from the shower floor, or reaching into the trunk of the car to pick up a grocery bag, is a big accomplishment to the individual who believes they cannot and might not ever be able to do them again. These activities all require integrated movement of the spine and extremities.[39] Worldwide, the prevalence of low back pain ranges from 30% to 83%, whereas people in wealthier countries like the United States have an even higher prevalence of low back pain. It is estimated that 25% to 60% of Americans who experience an episode of low back pain lasting longer than 1 year will continue to have chronic and reoccurring low back pain for the rest of their life.[40] This translates into an estimated $280 billion a year in health care costs in the United States alone.[39-41] Our health care systems are overwhelmed because of the lack of control we have over the incidence of chronic pain and the effect they have on our society, economy, and overall well-being. There are many factors including positive, pain-free movement experiences that can significantly shift the beliefs and perceptions related to pain and movement. New movement strategies and positive experiences can greatly improve the psychosocial limitations we experience on a daily basis.[37,38] We also know that when people who believe they cannot move finally have an opportunity to move without pain, they will experience a paradigm shift that affects their perceived quality of life for the better.[37,38,42-44]

BIOENERGETICS

Mobility of the spine and all the body is important for the flow of life's energy or prana. With an increase in flowing and controlled movement, we can theoretically expect to experience stronger immune systems, improved digestion, improved circulation, and regulated blood pressure capable of distributing blood through the entire body.[23,45-47]

CONCLUSION

The mobility of joints, noncontractile tissues (including ligaments, cartilage, capsules, discs, and labra), contractile tissues (myofascial), and nervous tissue are essential for successful movement. When one experiences structural restrictions in any of these tissues, mobility will need to occur somewhere else and may be less efficient. This compensation strategy could be necessary in the case of a fusion or severe scar tissue. Most times there is enough redundancy in the human body to accomplish most of our daily tasks naturally, easily, and spontaneously with these compensations. Mobility is necessary to have control of movement; otherwise, we merely experience rigidity. In the following chapters, the principles of alignment, control, and movement integration are discussed. The following questions are answered in the next chapter: How does our neuromuscular control match our available mobility? What happens when we do not have control over the mobility in our tissues? How does this compare to what happens when we do not have enough mobility for the desired task? and How might the neuromuscular system compensate for a loss of mobility in a region of the body? I believe as we ask these questions, light bulbs begin to light up our understanding of how the body moves.

OPEN-ENDED QUESTIONS

1 Explain in your own words how mobility is required before the body can express control.

2 Describe "the distribution of movement equals the distribution of force" in your own words.

3 How might restoration of movement of a neighboring joint affect the affected joint identified with dysfunction? How might this strategy be used in movement education?

4 What defines global muscles? What effect do global muscles have on the axial skeleton?

5 What defines local muscles? What effect do local muscles have on the axial skeleton?

6 Expand on the application of the term *bandha* according to Simon Borg-Olivier's definition of a cocontraction of a joint complex. How can you apply the image to the balance of mobility and control of a joint complex?

7 How do noncontractile tissues of the body contribute to mobility? Give examples of how hypermobility and hypomobility of these structures can impair movement.

8 Demonstrate spine movement as it pertains to the orientation of the facet joints. Notice the different biases of the different regions of the spine. What region of the spine is most adept to rotational activities? Why? Repeat the same for flexion/extension bias and lateral flexion bias.

9 How can movement education greatly reduce unnecessary tissue stressors with normal recreational activities? Identify abnormal strategies and then replace them with more efficient strategies.

10 Explain, as if talking to a sedentary client/person, why they might need to spend extra time conditioning their tissues to tolerate movement in planes other than sagittal.

11 How does tissue adaptation learn to respond correctly to new movement stressors? How do we know when the tissue has adapted sufficiently to sustain additional range, speed, and load?

12 Describe in your own words the planes of movement and load distribution for each of the lower extremity joints, and how they might contribute to efficiency of movement in their respective planes. Which joints complement each other with more complex movements like a swing of a tennis racquet or kicking a soccer ball?

13 Which lower extremity joints might compensate for a lack of ankle dorsiflexion? How might you assess if the restricted ankle dorsiflexion truly has a negative effect on other lower extremity joints and tissues?

OPEN-ENDED QUESTIONS

14 Describe in your own words the arthrokinematics of the knee while squatting. Sing out the spiral, spin, and glide directions of the femoral condyles.

15 Use the analogy of the jar opening to describe to someone the accessory motion in a joint as taught in arthrokinematics. What happens to the alignment when the lid and the jar move in the same direction? Can you extrapolate this analogy to faulty movement?

16 Describe the relationship between the thoracic cage, scapulae, and upper extremities with overhead activities. How can one maintain distribution of mobility in the glenohumeral joint when performing overhead activities (ie, spiking a volleyball)?

17 Identify commonalities and differences between the upper and lower extremities as they relate to function, weight-bearing, dexterity, and transfer/absorption of external forces. How can you apply their similarities and differences to fully integrated movement (ie, swimming, golfing, pitching, cross-country skiing)?

18 In many movement forms and conditioning, we are asked to weight-bear on our upper extremities. How would you teach an individual with hypermobility of noncontractile tissues of the upper extremity to do a plank or push-up? What might they find the most challenging? Where do you think the whole body connection takes place? Try it yourself and explore organizing the movement from the axial skeleton and working out and visa versa. How would you teach the plank to a novice? How do you progress toward efficiency?

19 What did you learn from the pilot study at Mount St. Mary's looking at distribution of movement in the thoracic and lumbar spine? How might you apply this information to a client who is suffering from mechanical low back pain at L5-S1? How would you explain the decreased back pain after doing Pilates?

20 In your own words, explain to a client or friend why their herniated lumbar disc no longer seems to be causing pain. How do you believe this can affect their beliefs about their pain?

REFERENCES

1. Pilates JH, Robbins J. *Pilates Evolution: The 21st Century.* Presentation Dynamics; 2012.
2. Vleeming A, Mooney V, Stoeckart R. *Movement, Stability & Lumbopelvic Pain: Integration of Research and Therapy.* 2nd ed. Churchill Livingstone; 2007.
3. Bogduk N, Twomey LT. *Clinical Anatomy of the Lumbar Spine.* Churchill Livingstone; 1987.
4. Colloca CJ, Keller TS, Moore RJ, Harrison DE, Gunzburg R. Validation of a noninvasive dynamic spinal stiffness assessment methodology in an animal model of intervertebral disc degeneration. *Spine (Phila Pa 1976).* 2009;34(18):1900-1905.
5. Nordin M, Frankel VH. *Basic Biomechanics of the Musculoskeletal System.* 2nd ed. Lea & Febiger; 1989.

6. Porterfield JA, DeRosa C. *Mechanical Low Back Pain: Perspectives in Functional Anatomy.* Saunders; 1991.

7. Harrison DE, Cailliet R, Harrison DD, Janik TJ. How do anterior/posterior translations of the thoracic cage affect the sagittal lumbar spine, pelvic tilt, and thoracic kyphosis? *Eur Spine J.* 2002;11(3):287-293.

8. Harrison DE, Colloca CJ, Harrison DD, Janik TJ, Haas JW, Keller TS. Anterior thoracic posture increases thoracolumbar disc loading. *Eur Spine J.* 2005;14(3):234-242.

9. Harrison DE, Janik TJ, Cailliet R, et al. Upright static pelvic posture as rotations and translations in 3-dimensional from three 2-dimensional digital images: validation of a computerized analysis. *J Manipulative Physiol Ther.* 2008;31(2):137-145.

10. Lee DG. Biomechanics of the thorax—research evidence and clinical expertise. *J Man Manip Ther.* 2015;23(3):128-138.

11. Bayliss J. *Spinal mechanics.* 2005. http://spinalmechanics.com/fryette.html

12. Panjabi MM, Brand RA Jr, White 3rd AA. Mechanical properties of the human thoracic spine as shown by three-deminesional load-displacement curves. *J Bone Joint Surg Am.* 1976;58(5):642-652.

13. Tsang SM, Szeto GP, Lee RY. Normal kinematics of the neck: the interplay between the cervical and thoracic spines. *Man Ther.* 2013;18(5):431-437.

14. Bergmark A. Stability of the lumbar spine. A study in mechanical engineering. *Acta Orthop Scand Suppl.* 1989;230:1-54.

15. Radzimińska A, Weber-Rajek M, Strączyńska A, Zukow W. The stabilizing system of the spine. *J Educ Health Sport.* 2017;7(11):67-76.

16. Black M, Calais-Germain B, Vleeming A. *Centered: Organizing the Body Through Kinesiology, Movement Theory and Pilates Technique.* Handspring Publishing; 2015.

17. Richardson C, Hodges PW, Hides J. *Therapeutic Exercise for Lumbo-Pelvic Stabilisation: A Motor Control Approach for the Treatment and Prevention of Low Back Pain.* 2nd ed. Churchill Livingstone; 2004.

18. Panjabi MM. The stabilizing system of the spine. Part II. Neutral zone and instability hypothesis. *J Spinal Disord.* 1992;5(4):390-396; discussion 397.

19. Panjabi MM. The stabilizing system of the spine. Part I. Function, dysfunction, adaptation, and enhancement. *J Spinal Disord.* 1992;5(4):383-389; discussion 397.

20. Sangwan S, Green RA, Taylor NF. Characteristics of stabilizer muscles: a systematic review. *Physiother Can.* 2014;66(4):348-358.

21. O'Sullivan PB, Twomey L, Allison GT. Altered abdominal muscle recruitment in patients with chronic back pain following a specific exercise intervention. *J Orthop Sports Phys Ther.* 1998;27(2):114-124.

22. O'Sullivan PB, Phyty GD, Twomey LT, Allison GT. Evaluation of specific stabilizing exercise in the treatment of chronic low back pain with radiologic diagnosis of spondylolysis or spondylolisthesis. *Spine (Phila Pa 1976).* 1997;22(24):2959-2967.

23. Borg-Olivier S. *Applied Anatomy & Physiology of Yoga.* Warisanoffset.com; 2006.

24. Hodges PW, Richardson CA. Inefficient muscular stabilization of the lumbar spine associated with low back pain: a motor control evaluation of transversus abdominis. *Spine (Phila Pa 1976).* 1996;21(22):2640-2650.

25. Bordoni B, Lintonbon D, Morabito B. Meaning of the solid and liquid fascia to reconsider the model of biotensegrity. *Cureus.* 2018;10(7):e2922.

26. Bordoni B, Simonelli M. The awareness of the fascial system. *Cureus.* 2018;10(10):e3397.

27. Fischer BM, Inge MM, Jenkins TM, Inge TH. Sitting time and long-term weight change in adolescents with severe obesity undergoing surgical and nonoperative weight management. *J Surg Obes Relat Dis.* 2020;16(3):431-436.

28. Loyen A, Chey T, Engelen L, et al. Recent trends in population levels and correlates of occupational and leisure sitting time in full-time employed Australian adults. *PLOS One.* 2018;13(4):e0195177.

29. Wolff's law. Wikipedia. Updated October 15, 2022. https://en.wikipedia.org/wiki/Wolff%27s_law

30. Schleip R, Baker A, Avison J. *Fascia in Sport and Movement.* Handspring Publishing; 2015.

31. Greenman PE. *Principles of Manual Medicine.* Williams and Wilkins; 1989.

32. Earls J. *Born to Walk: Myofascial Efficiency and the Body in Movement.* North Atlantic Books; 2014.

33. Earls J, Myers TW. *Fascial Release for Structural Balance.* North Atlantic Books; 2010.

34. Myers TW. *Anatomy Trains: Myofascial Meridians for Manual and Movement Therapists.* 3rd ed. Elsevier; 2014.

35. Franklin EN. *Conditioning for Dance.* Human Kinetics; 2004.

36. Schleip R. *Fascia: The Tensional Network of the Human Body: The Science and Clinical Applications in Manual and Movement Therapy.* Churchill Livingstone/Elsevier; 2012.

37. Lackner JM, Carosella AM. The relative influence of perceived pain control, anxiety, and functional self efficacy on spinal function among patients with chronic low back pain. *Spine (Phila Pa 1976).* 1999;24(21):2254-2260; discussion 2260-2251.

38. Anderson BD. *Randomized Clinical Trial Comparing Active Versus Passive Approaches to the Treatment of Recurrent and Chronic Low Back Pain* [dissertation]. University of Miami; 2005.

39. Fatoye F, Gebrye T, Odeyemi I. Real-world incidence and prevalence of low back pain using routinely collected data. *Rheumatol Int.* 2019;39(4):619-626.

40. Manchikanti L, Singh V, Datta S, Cohen SP, Hirsch JA, American Society of International Pain Physicians. Comprehensive review of epidemiology, scope, and impact of spinal pain. *Pain Physician.* 2009;12(4):E35-E70.

41. Dagenais S, Caro J, Haldeman S. A systematic review of low back pain cost of illness studies in the United States and internationally. *Spine J.* 2008;8(1):8-20.

42. Mannion AF, Junge A, Taimela S, Muntener M, Lorenzo K, Dvorak J. Active therapy for chronic low back pain: part 3. Factors influencing self-rated disability and its change following therapy. *Spine (Phila Pa 1976).* 2001;26(8):920-929.

43. Mannion AF, Taimela S, Muntener M, Dvorak J. Active therapy for chronic low back pain part 1. Effects on back muscle activation, fatigability, and strength. *Spine (Phila Pa 1976).* 2001;26(8):897-908.

44. Priebe S, Savill M, Reininghaus U, et al. Effectiveness and cost-effectiveness of body psychotherapy in the treatment of negative symptoms of schizophrenia—a multi-centre randomised controlled trial. *BMC Psychiatry.* 2013;13:26.

45. Feuerstein G. *The Shambhala Guide to Yoga.* 1st ed. Shambhala; 1996.

46. Hewitt J. *The Complete Yoga Book: Yoga of Breathing, Yoga of Posture, and Yoga of Meditation.* Schocken Books; 1978.

47. Yogananda. *Autobiography of a Yogi.* Crystal Clarity Publishers; 1946.

ALIGNMENT

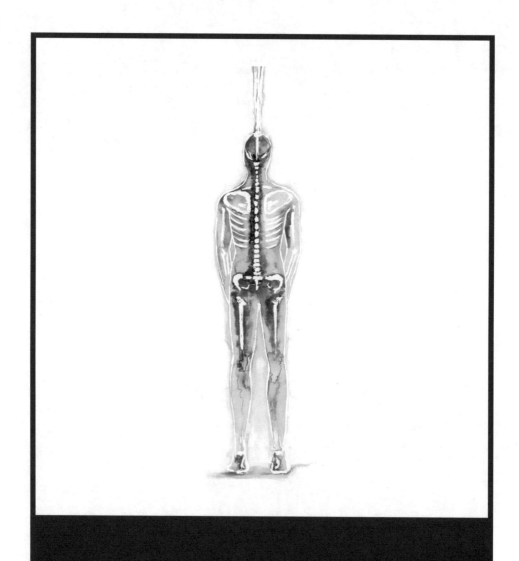

FOCUS ON ALIGNMENT AND LOAD, AND TRUST THE BODY WILL LEARN.

CHAPTER OBJECTIVES

1 Understand the effect alignment and joint congruence have on the neuromuscular system's ability to organize complex spontaneous movements.

2 Use dynamic alignment as one of the main tools to assess an individual's movement effectiveness.

3 Differentiate between static and dynamic alignment as they relate to functional movements.

4 Appreciate how our posture can affect the visual, auditory, and proprioceptive structures in the head and body.

5 Develop the practitioner's eyes to observe the mover and their ability to maintain optimal congruency of the joints throughout the task or activity.

6 Incorporate Manohar Panjabi's model of central neural control, contractile structures, and noncontractile structures to optimize movement efficiency and dynamic alignment.

KEY TERMS
- Alignment
- Axial elongation
- Congruence
- Dynamic
- Gait
- Panjabi's model
- Spontaneous
- Static

With ample mobility in the body's joints and soft tissues required for the desired level of activity and participation, dynamic alignment can be used to facilitate spontaneous and efficient neuromuscular organization for the desired movement. This is the principle of alignment. When a human's posture is correctly aligned, load creates the messaging to spontaneously engage the neuromuscular and fascial systems to sustain, propel, decelerate, and move in all planes for the desired movement. In Polestar, we use alignment and load as powerful tools to facilitate proper neuromuscular activation without having to use isolated muscle contraction cueing. The challenge is understanding human anatomy and arthrokinematics well enough to know that the body is dynamically congruent and aligned through the movement sequence. Alignment combined with a graded load can gradually educate the body in a natural and childlike way to restore healthy human movement.

FOCUS ON ALIGNMENT AND LOAD, AND TRUST THE BODY WILL LEARN.

The 3rd principle, alignment, is one of my favorite principles. The word alignment is probably the most important and beneficial word that we can use to improve and enhance the quality of our life and our movement. Interestingly, alignment is not limited to the physical body; it expands to mental, spiritual, and social aspects of us as well.

Anderson BD.
Principles of Movement (pp 98-123).
© 2024 Taylor & Francis Group.

How do we as movement practitioners facilitate the alignment between our perception and reality? Alignment is necessary for self-fulfillment; Abraham Maslow explains it in his hierarchy of the human needs. Before self-actualization, we need to be aligned. Therefore, repeatedly what we do as movement practitioners is much more than just teach exercises. We reinforce self-esteem, confidence, and alignment. When people experience physical alignment of their bodies, they experience emotional, mental, and spiritual alignment as well. They are inseparable.

Although there are many who have not experienced a sense of connection between mind, body, and spirit, after a thoughtful movement session, you will hear things, such as "I cannot believe how happy I am when I am consistent with my yoga or Pilates" and "I cannot believe how much clearer my head is when I run 5 days a week." We hear these types of testimonials repeatedly. It makes sense. We study the body and understand that when our musculoskeletal system is balanced, the other systems, including the digestion, immune, circulatory, and nervous systems, all function better. When our systems function better, our mind is clearer. We tend to think better, and we tend to perform better at work. We tend to be happier, and we tend to be kinder. We see things as being more beautiful in the world. Alignment is everything. Let us move into the anatomical aspect of our physical body and how the knowledge of the anatomy can facilitate better alignment of all aspects of the human being.

Eric Franklin defined ideal alignment as follows: "… all the body parts approximating toward the central axis as much as structure permits." The beauty of Franklin's phrase is "as much as structure permits."[1] A patient of mine has scoliosis. If she organizes her structure toward the central axis, as much as her structure permits, she will experience her ideal alignment in that moment.

No longer should we try to define everyone by where they fit in the old Florence Peterson Kendall and Elizabeth Kendall McCreary charts of ideal postures when we used to say "This is what perfect posture is" or "This is what you have to look like." Rather, how do we get our bodies to perform at their optimal potential?

BOX 5-1

Years ago, I was out waterskiing with some friends of mine. I was thinking that I was "all that" and "laying it down." In my mind, I thought that I was shooting up a very big spray of water as my body angled inches from the water. My impression was that I was matching what my much more skilled friends looked like as they skied. However, as I was taking off my Connelly HP Slalom ski, my friend John said, "Hey Brent, you really suck at waterskiing." Of course my ego did not allow me to believe that, so I challenged his remark and said, "Prove it." John had a smile on his face as he showed me a video he had taken of me skiing that day. I looked like I was shaking and making a quick release movement that was not fluid, and my body was more vertical than horizontal—an amateur performance compared to my friends. I realized that I was not aligned. By this, I mean that my perception of my movement was nowhere close to the reality of my movement.

ALIGNMENT OF THE AXIAL SKELETON

We are the only mammal that has a bicurve spine (see Figure 4-28 in Chapter 4). That means we have a lordotic curve in our lumbar spine and a kyphotic curve in our thoracic spine. This allows us to be upright, bipedal animals that can walk and run without falling over. These curves are unique even from our close relatives, the primates, who have a continuous curve from the sacrum all the way up to the cervical spine. The human's bicurve spine allows us the ability to be upright all the time and to have increased dexterity of our upper extremities. If we lose the axial length in our spines, we start to lose function in our desired movement. Our sedentary lives are challenging our bicurve spine. We frequently see people with poor posture and subsequently compromised movement strategies. If you sit slouched forward and try to lift your arms up over your head or turn your head to the right and left, you will notice a significant loss of range and ease of what should be a natural movement. Now sit tall. As you lift your arms up or move your head right to left, you will notice more range of motion just by placing the spine in a more elongated or optimal posture.

In each of the vertebral segments, there is a weight-bearing disc between the vertebral bodies anterior to the spinal canal and the zygapophyseal (facet) joints (see Figures 4-15A and 4-15B in Chapter 4). This is referred to as the *tripod weight-bearing structure*.[2] Balanced weight-bearing between the disc and the facets aligns the axial skeleton so it is closer to the central axis, resulting in greater axial length, or what we refer to as *axial elongation*. How do we obtain axial elongation? What exactly is it? Imagine your spine in the presence of gravity being compressed, exaggerating the curves. Axial elongation of the axial skeleton is the opposite; it is a gentle lengthening that restores the healthy spinal curves. It is an optimal position or alignment that allows us

to move more efficiently and with greater ease. When the vertebral segments are optimally aligned, we have the greatest degrees of freedom in all planes of movement (ie, flexion, extension, lateral flexion, rotation, circumduction, and combined planes). This enhances the ability to perform complex movements with decreased load distributed through many segments instead of only a few. Think of how many motions of the spine there are in a tennis serve. When potential movement options are removed because of poor habitual posture (eg, slouching), we lose available mobility. Now imagine someone playing tennis with a slouched posture and related loss of shoulder flexion and cervical rotation as we experienced in the arm-raising exercise described earlier. Where would the movement come from with little to no mobility in the thoracic spine and hips, which are both primary sources of rotation in a tennis serve? The force of the movement will be biased to the shoulder joint, knees, or the low back; that tennis player theoretically might end up with shoulder, knee, or back injuries because they did not access the mobility in their thoracic spine and hips. Optimization of alignment becomes a primary focus in the assessment of the individual and their ability to participate in the activities they choose. According to Bordoni et al[3,4] and the biotensegrity model, the axial structures are stabilized by the balance of constant tension and the presence of a discontinuous compression. This organization is self-stabilizing, allowing it to manage tension variations with a certain degree of flexibility and transferring the forces applied to the whole structure.[3,4] This model can also be explained by the Golgi organ receptors found in the fascia, which are responsible for upright posture. When tension is balanced around the axial skeleton, the performance of contractile and noncontractile tissues exponentially becomes more efficient. Joseph Pilates stated, "Good posture can only be successfully acquired when the entire mechanism of the body is under perfect control. Graceful carriage follows as a matter of course."[5] Joseph Pilates innately understood how powerful good postural control is when maintained throughout our daily life. He was even quoted in *Reader's Digest* as saying, "You're walking along the street. Glance in the shop window, not to lower your sales resistance, but to observe your own posture. Most [people] use the shop windows as mirrors anyway—but merely to see if their hats are on straight rather than if their heads are on straight."[6] This idea of optimal dynamic posture is a good place to start in our explanation of axial elongation.

Alignment of the axial skeleton plays a major role in our spatial awareness. Another important aspect of alignment is how our senses and proprioception provide feedback for successful movement and dynamic alignment. The head houses many of the structures we use for balance and spatial awareness, including the inner ear, eyes, and cerebellum. The position of the head is crucial for the vestibular system to work efficiently. If the head is not able to orient the eyes and the semicircular canals correctly, then the information coming into the central nervous system will be erroneous and confusing. The righting reflexes and the vestibulo-ocular reflexes are interdependent with accurate head orientation. The reticular formation is a series of tracts responsible for maintaining tone, balance, and posture, especially during body movements. The reticular formation also relays eye and ear signals to the cerebellum, so the cerebellum can integrate visual, auditory, and vestibular stimuli in motor coordination. All the proprioceptive input is thought to be coordinated here. The deep local stabilizers of the head and neck can provide that proprioceptive information when they are not compromised by poor posture.[7,8] Another great source of postural feedback is in the spine's noncontractile structures, including the ligaments, capsules, discs, and bones.

When the head is aligned well, sensory coordination is thought to be optimized. Senses such as sight, sound, taste, and smell appear to be experienced more fully when the head and neck are well aligned. Clinically, I have noticed that when patients regain their head posture, they will experience heightened senses.

ESSENTIAL SCIENCES
NONCONTRACTILE STRUCTURES OF THE AXIAL SKELETON

The noncontractile structures of the cervical, thoracic, and lumbar spine play a major role in the alignment and control of the axial skeleton. Ligaments are made up primarily of collagen fibers, like the annulus of the disc. The collagen fibers create stiffness. They hold the bones together. Their job is to avoid excessive movement within a joint. Inside of these ligaments are mechanoreceptors that tell us when there is load or tension. When we move our spine in a different direction and we get close to the end of that range of motion, a message is sent to the central nervous system saying that we are approaching an end of range. These messages stimulate a protective reflex to maintain stability in that joint through neuromuscular cocontraction.

The anterior longitudinal ligament is a very thick ligament in the front of our spine (Figure 5-1). This ligament provides an anterior reinforcement to the lordotic nature of the lumbar spine. It protects against anterior shear force between the vertebrae. Some people have a spinal defect or have injured the anterior longitudinal ligament, which might lead to spondylolisthesis (Figure 5-2). In spondylolisthesis, the superior vertebra is anteriorly displaced on the inferior vertebrae. The anterior displacement can result in stenosis of the transverse foramen, as well as the central foramen, because of a laxity of the anterior longitudinal ligament.

Just behind the vertebral bodies is the posterior longitudinal ligament (see Figure 4-13 in Chapter 4). The posterior longitudinal ligament is much thinner and narrower than the anterior longitudinal ligament. As bipedal animals, there is less stress on the posterior column ligament, especially in the lumbar spine. Over the past 100 years, we have become more

ANTERIOR VIEW

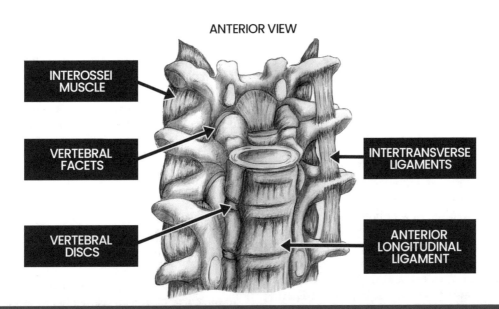

INTEROSSEI MUSCLE

VERTEBRAL FACETS

VERTEBRAL DISCS

INTERTRANSVERSE LIGAMENTS

ANTERIOR LONGITUDINAL LIGAMENT

Figure 5-1. The anterior longitudinal ligament.   (Illustrated by Kelly Anderson.)

sedentary than ever. When we sit for long periods of time, we flex our lumbar spine, all without the same protection that the anterior longitudinal ligament gives the anterior spine. Because of this, the posterior annulus fibers of the disc are exposed to prolonged stresses. It will be interesting to see in our next evolution if the posterior longitudinal ligament begins to look more like the anterior longitudinal ligament to support our flexed spines in sitting. Most of our disc injuries are thought to be a result of prolonged flexion activities and sedentarism rather than accidents, and the solution is more movement and less prolonged sitting.

The ligamentum flavum, as discussed in Chapter 4 (see Figure 4-13), is more elastic and serves to help maintain axial elongation of the axial skeleton. I like to use the image of the ligamentum flavum to ease into the restoring of uprightness from a flexed spine posture. An elastic band can be used to simulate the ligamentum flavum by stretching the band from the top of the head to the tailbone in standing; then, flex the spine forward, and feel the elastic effect from the band wanting to return the body to its upright posture. Next, take the

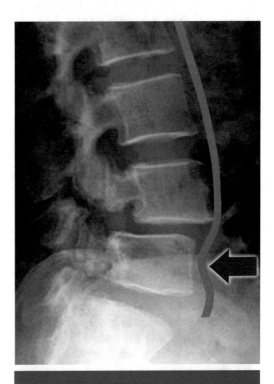

Figure 5-2. X-ray showing spondylolisthesis (blue arrow).

(Illustrated by Kelly Anderson.)

band away, and see if the image can continue to facilitate an effortless segmental stacking of the vertebrae into a vertical posture.

The ligaments surrounding the sacroiliac joints (SIJs) and lumbopelvic region are extensive and very thick (see Figures 4-2A and 4-2B in Chapter 4). It is important to note that the manual therapy literature often depicts the SIJ as a mobile joint, whereas anatomists describe it as an immobile joint. I believe it is somewhere in the middle, but I lean toward the anatomists' view of immobility. The L5-S1 segment lines up horizontally with the SIJ and is much more likely to be mobile. Occasionally, I have seen a true sacroiliac sprain caused by a severe car accident or during pregnancy when the ligaments are loosening and preparing for partum, but typically they are so strong that the pelvic bone will fracture before the ligaments deform. Think of them like a suspension system in a sports car. If I am in a hot Porsche and driving around a curve fast, the suspension plates below absorb the force of the curve and push the tire and suspension back into the ground so that I do not feel the sway. However, if I am driving an old van with a very poor suspension system and I am coming around a curve faster than 20 mph/32 kph, I feel a tremendous amount of sway to the side. It is not absorbing the potential energy. I think of our pelvis as being like a Porsche suspension system. When our bones are aligned correctly, the potential energy is absorbed from the ground in these ligaments and bones and either returned to the ground as an accelerating or elastic energy or dispersed through the rest of the body. This is a very powerful concept pertaining to moving efficiently, comparing elasticity with muscle contraction. We have noticed that elite runners use very little muscle energy while running. I believe there will be an increase in the body of knowledge showing how the myofascial system combined with proper alignment and load will become the primary focus of conditioning with a focus on tissue adaptation for tissues to be more elastic in nature.

As discussed previously, the discs of the spine are essential noncontractile structures that obtain and maintain dynamic alignment. The mobility of the discs in all planes and their ability to hydrate through movement in a healthy mobile spine can greatly reduce unwanted forces and improve the natural strategy to maintain an axially elongated spine through all combinations of movement (Box 5-2).

ALIGNMENT OF THE LOWER EXTREMITY

The angle of the sacrum is closely related to the curve of our lumbar spine. In terms of axial elongation, we must also align the sacrum to its neighboring lumbar vertebra above and the pelvis in relationship to the femur below (Figure 5-3). Ideally, the innominate or pelvic half should rest vertically on the head of the femur in an upright position. You can see the femur is angled, and the head of the femur moves inward into the pelvis. In standing, the heads of the femurs should line up vertically with the ankles. You can also notice the proximity of the vertical line between the ala area of the sacrum and the head of the femur. This is another unique anatomical trait of humans compared with primates.[9] This allows for minimal lateral shift of the pelvis to maintain optimal vertical alignment on top of the lower extremity when standing, walking, running, and jumping. Imagine the spine and pelvis in their axial orientation and the connective tissue weaving through and in between as tensile force generators. These myofascial fibers can provide stiffness, elasticity, acceleration, and deceleration depending on the bony alignment in relationship to gravity, momentum, and the desired movement outcome.

BOX 5-2: HYDRATION TIP

1. Hydrate by drinking plenty of water.
2. Avoid drinks and foods that dehydrate (eg, alcohol, coffee, and caffeinated drinks).
3. Smoking tobacco is a major cause of disc degeneration and dehydration. STOP!
4. Segmental movement is a hydrator of the discs and can also remove waste. Try the following basic to more challenging movements to keep your discs healthy:
   a. Pelvic clock supine and sitting
   b. Bridging with articulation
   c. Bridging with lateral translation and diagonals
   d. Controlled movements in all planes in standing (eg, standing roll down, standing saw)
   e. Dancing

ALIGNMENT OF THE HEAD AND UPPER EXTREMITY

The upper extremities and the head are significant differentiators of the human being from most other animals. Our ability to sense the environment and interact with the dexterity necessary to manipulate and execute tasks with our hands has made humans very powerful in the animal kingdom. The head, neck, and shoulders are also good indicators of energy expenditure. It is quite common to see elevated shoulders, clenched teeth, and squinting eyes when someone is acquiring a new movement. I like to think that a great benefit of applying this principle, in addition to many great benefits, is that the head, neck, and shoulders act like the eyes into the soul of efficient movement organization. We can use the organization of the head, neck, and shoulders to understand where our clients are in the learning of new tasks and the improvement of faulty strategies of old tasks.

Think back to the first time you learned to ride a bike. As you grabbed your handlebars, your shoulders were up around your ears and your arms locked and shaking. You were over-recruiting muscles, and you were getting in your own way. After a couple weeks

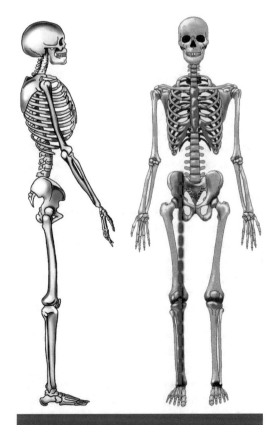

Figure 5-3. The lateral and anterior view of the skeleton. Axial alignment of the pelvis, hip, knee, and foot.

of riding the bike, you got to the point where you could relax and even take your hands off the handlebars—"Look, no hands!" This over-recruitment is obvious by the clenching of the jaw, the raising of the shoulders, and working hard to "get it," which are all signs of novice movement organization.

The organization of the head, neck, and shoulders is a valuable tool for assessing an individual's alignment and movement efficiency. We can better understand the role of the head, neck, and shoulders by deepening our understanding of the anatomy and biomechanics of these regions of the body. Remember that many of the balance centers reside in the head, including the vestibular system, vision, and the center for proprioception, as previously discussed.

ANATOMY OF THE HEAD, NECK, AND SHOULDERS

I remember years ago doing a study with some dentists and physical therapists who treated temporomandibular dysfunction. The interventions were special splints or prosthetics to minimize bruxing (ie, grinding the teeth) and optimize the alignment of the temporomandibular joint (TMJ). By accident, we discovered that after fitting patients with their prosthesis to unload their bite, there was a secondary effect of a temporary improvement of musculoskeletal alignment issues, such as scoliosis, pelvic torsion, and shoulder asymmetries. How and why would that happen? We realized that the TMJ is a powerful balance center in the body.

The TMJs are located just in front of the inner ear where the vestibular system is located (Figure 5-4). It is important to repeat that when the head is in ideal posture, and all the circular canals and visual fields are organized most accurately with gravity and the environment, chewing and talking are biomechanically more efficient. Good posture goes far beyond just looking good in front of the mirror or in a selfie.

The hyoid bone is a small bone in the front of the throat; it is suspended with the strap muscles, which attach to it from above and below. The hyoid moves up and down as part of the swallowing mechanism, aiding in the ability to move food to the digestive system and to facilitate air exchange. When the head and neck are poorly aligned, swallowing and breathing are labored. I always think of the patients I saw when working in the hospital and the difficulty they had eating and breathing. I remember the position of their head and neck while in a hospital bed. This could be an easy fix if we had simply propped them up differently.

The cervical spine anatomy was previously discussed in the mobility principle in Chapter 4; it is important to remember that it should have a lordotic curve, and its primary purpose is to support the head and move the head to sense the environment. In this chapter, I want to draw your attention more toward the relationship between the head and the first 2 cervical vertebrae. In Figure 4-8 in Chapter 4, observe how C1 and C2 are completely horizontal in their relationship to the occiput of the head and gravity. The atlanto-occipital joint

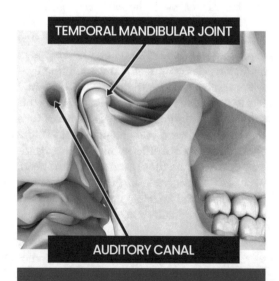

TEMPORAL MANDIBULAR JOINT

AUDITORY CANAL

Figure 5-4. The TMJ.
(Alex Mitt/Shutterstock.com.)

allows 50% of the flexion and extension of the head and 50% of the side flexion of the head. The next segment down is C1-2. It is here that 50% of the head's rotation occurs or should occur. Today, the head, neck, and shoulders are often rounded forward, placing the suboccipital region in terminal extension and leaving very little motion in the suboccipital region for rotation or extension (Figures 5-5A and 5-5B) because the spine has moved as far as it can in this direction. Let us imagine what might happen to the head, jaw, and cervical spine if someone with poor driving posture was rear-ended. The TMJ is in an unstable position and will be thrust forward, resulting in unnecessary damage to the TMJ ligaments and disc. Because the suboccipital region is locked up and not mobile, the forces will transfer down the cervical spine, and the bulk of the force will translate through C4-7, resulting in a whiplash injury. It would take a much stronger force to do the same damage if the joints were in proper orientation with gravity and in an axially elongated posture; the person would be much more resilient.

Moving into the alignment of the shoulder girdle, the scapulothoracic joint is aligned through a neuromuscular orchestra and absent of noncontractile structures as found in all other joints of the body. The muscles that connect the scapula to the trunk consist of the rhomboid major and minor, and they retract the scapula toward the spine (see Figure 4-35 in Chapter 4). The trapezius, the very large flat muscle that connects the scapula to the base of the head and inferiorly to the spinous processes in the cervical and thoracic spine all the way to T12, aids in upward and downward rotation of the scapulae (see Figure 4-41A in Chapter 4). The latissimus dorsi connects on the inferior slip of the scapulae and aids in downward rotation or resists upward rotation. The latissimus dorsi fascia melds with the thoracolumbar fascia and is part of the posterior diagonal fascial slings.[10,11] Anteriorly, the pectoralis minor originates from the coracoid process of the scapula and attaches to the superior medial ribs. The pectoralis minor provides a downward rotation moment and protracts the scapula (see Figure 4-41B in Chapter 4). The levator scapulae muscle originates from the superior angle of the scapula and inserts like

[A]
FORWARD HEAD

[B]
NEUTRAL ALIGNMENT

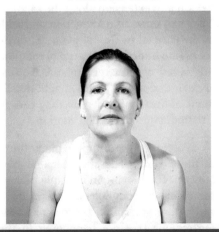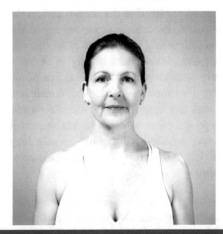

Figure 5-5. (A) A forward head places the suboccipital region in hyperextension. (B) Neutral alignment of the head.

fingers into the cervical vertebrae (see Figure 4-41B in Chapter 4). The serratus anterior attaches from the anterior medial surface of the scapulae, and its fingers insert into the lateral rib cage, drawing the scapulae into protraction (see Figures 4-36 and 4-41A in Chapter 4). I mentioned earlier that the muscles connecting the scapula to the torso are like a springy spiderweb or a trampoline. The tension from these muscles synergistically allows the scapula to be in alignment with the humerus and provides a distribution of force into the torso. The scapula and the humerus need to work together to maintain good alignment and congruence. If the scapula is winging or unable to move into extension and axial rotation, then the force will be absorbed in the glenohumeral joint or other joints in the upper extremity (eg, the elbow or wrist). Many upper extremity aches and pains can be relieved with proper alignment of the shoulder joint, maintenance of the shoulder blade against the ribs, and good thoracic mobility.

The next set of muscles connect the scapula to the humerus. This includes the supraspinatus, infraspinatus, subscapularis, and teres minor, also known collectively as the *rotator cuff* (see Figures 4-37A and 4-37B in Chapter 4). The rotator cuff muscles, when isolated, can externally and internally rotate the humerus, but collectively and more functionally, they approximate the head of the humerus into the glenoid fossa, increasing congruence of the joint and enhancing the efficiency of the surrounding muscles and the ability to respond efficiently to momentum acting on the upper extremity. The teres major, deltoid, coracobrachialis, and the long heads of the biceps and the triceps are often referred to as the *movers of the upper extremity*. They are mostly long muscles that create direction and momentum of the arm.

The last grouping of muscles that connect the humerus to the thorax are responsible for acceleration and deceleration of the arm through space. They consist of the pectoralis major, which connects from just underneath the arm to the anterior rib cage, and the latissimus dorsi (discussed earlier), which connects from the arm to the ribs in the back and down into the thoracolumbar fascia. These muscles are oriented in a diagonal orientation toward the center of the body (the latissimus posteriorly and the pectoralis major anteriorly). The pectoralis major is in the same diagonal as the opposite internal oblique muscle, and the latissimus dorsi is aligned with the gluteus maximus on the opposite side. These diagonal lines of muscles represent fascial chains that are part of a complex set of myofascial connections throughout the body that support and provide the elastic efficiencies of movement in the upright human body.[10-15]

BIOMECHANICS

In this section, the biomechanics of the upper and lower extremity joints are discussed, comparing them with their respective joints in the upper and lower extremity as it pertains to alignment and congruence.

THE HIP AND SHOULDER

The shoulder and hip are both ball-and-socket joints. They have 6 degrees of freedom (Figures 5-6A and 5-6B). They can move into flexion and extension along the sagittal plane. They can move into abduction and adduction in the coronal or frontal plane. They can also move into internal and external rotation in the horizontal or transverse plane. Because they are ball-and-socket joints, an additional movement of these joints is that they can perform circumduction or circular motion.

We rarely perform pure planar movement in these joints. The shoulder and hip joints are typically moving in multiple planes at the same time. For example, when I push a grocery cart, there are spiral, flexion, and extension movements that are happening in the ball-and-socket joints all at once. When we look at the muscles, we ask "Which muscle was responsible for this?" It might be that I was

[A]
SHOULDER JOINT

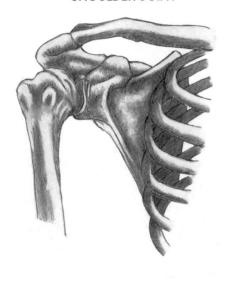

[B]
HIP JOINT

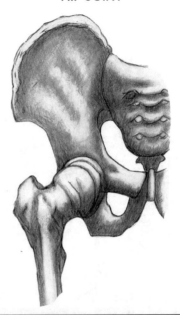

Figure 5-6. Ball-and-socket joints: (A) the shoulder joint and (B) the hip joint.
(Illustrated by Kelly Anderson.)

pushing the cart and my triceps were doing some pushing by lengthening my elbow, but the deceleration from my biceps and the spiral from my forearm were all part of managing how smoothly I pushed that cart. I find the relationship between the bones and their spatial reference to be one of the most important things to observe. When there is optimal alignment and congruence both in the extremities and the torso, the body has its greatest potential of natural and efficient movement. I choose the word "potential" carefully because the reality of achieving natural and efficient movement with our activities depends on our ability to practice and repeat the movement correctly enough times that the desired activity becomes spontaneous, and the neuromyofascial system efficiently maintains joint congruence and alignment.

THE KNEE AND ELBOW

The knee and elbow are the next joints in the kinetic chain of the extremities. Notice that both joints are hinge joints (Figures 5-8A and 5-8B). As mentioned earlier, the humeroulnar joint is a true hinge joint and only articulates in the sagittal plane. There is very little accessory joint motion or twisting in the elbow joint. On the other hand, the knee is a bicondylar joint, has rotation, and does have accessory joint motion beyond pure flexion and extension and rotation. I get very excited when I discuss the knee and how it affects the entire lower kinetic chain. The nature of this bicondylar joint is particularly interesting because the long femur bone angles toward midline at the knee, which is essential for single-leg weight-bearing. Because the medial condyle is significantly larger than the lateral condyle, it allows us to balance over the central

[A]

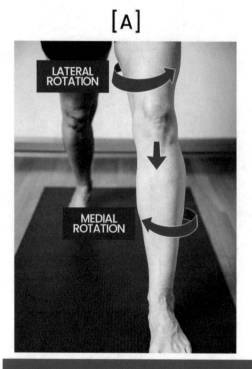

LATERAL
ROTATION

MEDIAL
ROTATION

[B]

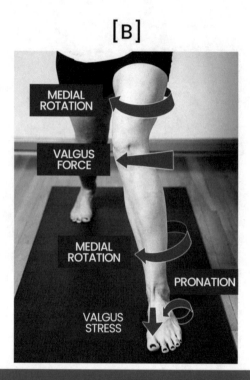

MEDIAL
ROTATION

VALGUS
FORCE

MEDIAL
ROTATION

PRONATION

VALGUS
STRESS

Figure 5-7. Heel strike during gait. (A) Normal alignment of lower extremity and (B) abnormal alignment of lower extremity, medially rotated hip, valgus knee, and pronated foot.

axis in single-leg weight-bearing (see Figures 4-20A and 4-20B in Chapter 4). The asymmetry between the medial and lateral condyles explains and facilitates the natural spiral in the lower kinetic chain that maintains alignment and stability during the load phase of walking or jumping. As mentioned previously, arthrokinematics refers to accessory motions, such as spin, glide, and spiral. In the dance medicine and movement science world, it is also referred to as *bone rhythms*. Eric Franklin explained that for years faulty movement patterns have been taught in the classical ballet world and have possibly been the culprit for traditional ballet-related injuries in the foot, ankle, knee, hip, and low back.[1] Arthrokinematically, in a squat, the femur will spiral laterally because the medial condyle is larger than the lateral. If the femur is spiraling laterally, then the tibia and the innominate or half of the pelvis spirals medially relative to the femur (Figure 5-7A). The result of this is lower extremity alignment,

power, and energy conservation. If the femur medially spirals during a squat, it will result in a loss of alignment, power, and efficiency. We can see the loss of alignment when both the femur and tibia medially rotate, resulting in valgus angle of the knees, eversion of the hindfoot, and prolonged pronation of the forefoot (Figure 5-7B). Further up the kinetic chain, we can see a possible anterior tilt of the pelvis, sacral nutation, and anterior shear force in the lumbar spine. It is impressive as a practitioner to work with someone who has been poorly taught or lost normal arthrokinematics because of injury. Simply correcting their movement pattern and bone rhythms can immediately influence a healthy neuromuscular strategy. As I mentioned in Chapter 1, I was treating a professional basketball player who had a series of left knee surgeries, the last of which was thought to have been very successful. Although this is what the doctors told him, the patient felt he still did not have the spring he was used to.

For him, it was not successful. In our first session, we spent about 30 minutes working on his arthrokinematics with assisted lunges on the Pilates chair where I guided the normal spiral patterns in his femur and tibia with my hands. It became obvious within minutes that this is what he was missing. He had plenty of strength, and his biomechanics had been restored by the surgery; he was just missing his normal accessory motions in the hip and knee. The following week he declared that he was back jumping like when he was in college.

As mentioned previously, the elbow, like the knee joint, is a hinge joint (see Figures 5-8A and 5-8B) but does not have the rotatory properties between the humerus and the ulna that exist in the lower extremity. We often refer to the humeroulnar joint as a *true hinge joint*.

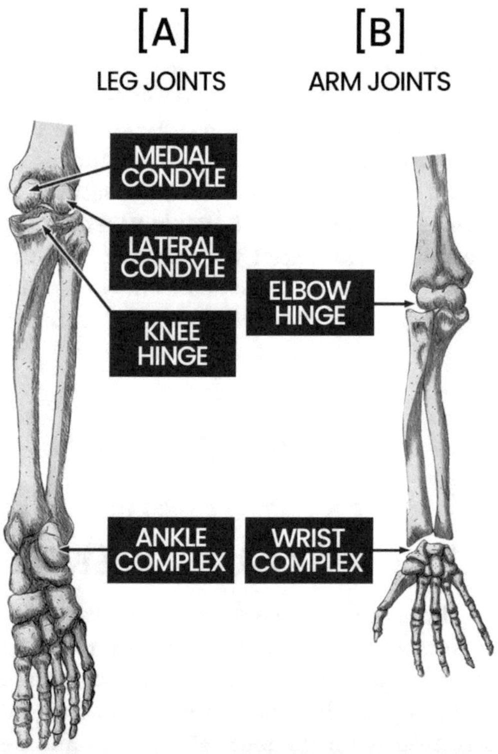

Figure 5-8. Hinge joints: (A) knee and ankle joints and (B) elbow and wrist joints.

(Illustrated by Kelly Anderson.)

Interestingly, the elbow is the most restricted joint by its bony nature and strong capsule and is limited to sagittal plane movement. In contrast, the joints above and below the elbow are extremely mobile and dexterous.

THE DISTAL LEG AND ARM

The biomechanics of the forearm, wrist, and hand allow for great dexterity. Our ability to manipulate objects for exploring, working, writing, eating, pushing, and pulling is often taken for granted. One of the unique biomechanical features of the forearm is the function of the radius in relationship to the humerus and the ulna and the proximal row of carpal bones (the wrist; see Figure 5-8B). Calais-Germain[16] discussed the unique shape of the radius and its movement properties, particularly to the curvature of the bone, which allows for the pronation and supination of the forearm where the radius rolls over the nonspiraling ulna. If the bones were straight and did not have differently shaped joints, they would not be able to pronate or supinate. These unique properties of the radius and ulna, differing from the lower leg anatomy, provide much more mobility and dexterity. In exchange for the dexterity of the upper extremity, we sacrifice some of the bony and ligamentous stability that we find in the lower extremity. Another unique feature of the radius is the articulation with the capitulum of the humerus. The round concave shape of the proximal radius and convex nature of the distal humerus create a ball-and-socket–like joint capable of flexion, extension, and rotation. Abduction or coronal plane movement is limited by the rigid sagittal plane movement of the humeroulnar joint. Lastly, the proximal radius is attached to the proximal ulna with the annular ligament, which, like a ring around the radius, facilitates its axial rotation. The distal radius articulates with the distal ulna where they make up a synovial joint and an articulating disc between the distal ulna and the proximal row of carpal bones. This will be important when we discuss closed- vs open-chain kinematics of the upper extremity.

The distal radius articulates with the proximal carpal bones and becomes the direct weight-bearing bone between the hand and the humerus, again uniquely different from the lower extremity in which the tibia is the primary weight-bearing and articulating bone between the talus and femur. The distal carpal bones articulate with the 5 metacarpal bones where the base of the metacarpal bone is concave and the head is convex, articulating with the proximal phalanges of the fingers. There is an interesting action that occurs when the metacarpophalangeal joints flex or extend. A passive adduction/abduction occurs to increase the stability of the wrist as we grasp tools or objects. This is a bit like the cocontraction that Simon Borg-Olivier discussed. A cocontraction around a joint complex, such as the wrist, will increase the stiffness to allow for the desired function. This can be seen when weight-bearing on the hand. If the metacarpophalangeal joints were to flex and the radiocarpal joints were extending, the tendons of these 2 muscle groups would create additional stability around the wrist when weight-bearing, called the *manibandha*[17] (Figure 5-9). The wrist is capable of movement in all planes where collectively the carpal bones with the distal radius and disc of the ulna create a ball-and-socket–like joint able to move in flexion/extension, adduction (ulnar deviation), abduction (radial deviation), and circumduction. The closed-packed position can be defined as the position in which there is maximum congruence of the articular surfaces, and joint stability is derived from the alignment of bones (eg, lifting the upper extremity to 90/90). In the wrist, the closed-packed position is in wrist extension and radial deviation; this is the most stable but is also vulnerable for injury. The functional hand position is where the wrist is in slight extension with radial deviation, the fingers are in slight flexion, and the thumb is abducted (see Figure 5-9). This results in a hollowed space under the palm of the hand. This movement will put your wrist into what we call a *safe space*. There is no way you can hang on your ligaments when you are in this position. The cocontraction between the flexors and extensors of your forearm will be working as a bandha in the upper extremity that will protect your wrist. Before you proceed with upper extremity weight-bearing exercises, make sure you are assessing your client's hands and wrists to make sure they are in the stable position as defined previously and not hyperextending their wrist. We do not want anyone to injure their wrist and be prevented from continuing their upper extremity weight-bearing training.

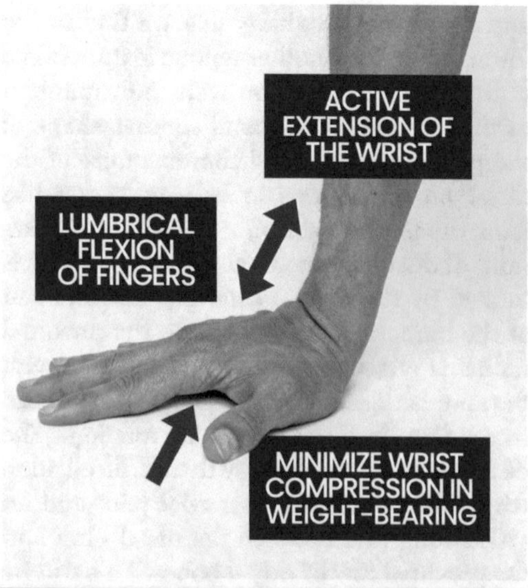

APPLICATION
STATIC VERSUS DYNAMIC ALIGNMENT

In contrast to the forearm, the lower leg is limited in its mobility between the tibia and fibula. The fibula glides superiorly and inferiorly and has little to no biomechanical properties with the femoral condyles and no real weight-bearing properties like the tibia. The fibula provides lateral stability because of its tendinous connection from the lateral hamstring tendons, the proximal synovial joint between the head of the fibula and the tibia,

ACTIVE EXTENSION OF THE WRIST

LUMBRICAL FLEXION OF FINGERS

MINIMIZE WRIST COMPRESSION IN WEIGHT–BEARING

Figure 5-9. Manibandha.

the interosseous membrane, and the distal syndesmosis between the fibula and the tibia. This distal union is not a true joint but rather a strong band of ligaments and fascia that control the lateral stability from the ankle all the way up into the origin of the lateral hamstring into the ischial tuberosity, contributing to the lateral and spiral lines according to Earls and Myers[10] and Myers.[11] It is important to note that the design of the upper extremity is not about weight-bearing but rather dexterity. In contrast, the lower extremity, although it has similar properties, is about weight-bearing and balance.

The ankle's biomechanics are unique as well and contribute significant mechanical properties for the bipedal nature of human locomotion. Many of us do not often think about the foot unless we stub a toe or get a blister, but we should because it is an amazingly adaptable and important structure. I often teach my patients that walking is controlled falling. Just by leaning forward as little as 5 degrees at the ankles, the foot and ankle are prepared, taut, and ready for launch. Mechanically, the talocrural joint becomes taut when the body weight is anterior of the vertical axis. The increased width of the anterior talus is responsible for the lever of the ankle and foot becoming stiff and preparing the body for propulsion and forward movement. The long levers of the body and muscle groups are responsible for controlled falling in which gravity is responsible for the forward movement and propulsion. Unfortunately, many clients weight-bear on the hindfoot, never achieving the proper amount of dorsiflexion in the ankle, which leaves the foot in pronation and does not stiffen the ankle and foot as a lever, resulting in a lack of natural mechanical propulsion and places undue stress on the connective tissues.

The alignment of the lower and upper extremities can vary greatly from individual to individual. There can also be a significant variance between static alignment and dynamic alignment. When we look at static posture and observe pronated feet, we might see knock-knees and hallux valgus (also known as a *bunion*), but, as mentioned previously, until we see the individual moving, we will not know how it affects their ability to move and whether it is structural malalignment or strategic misalignment. We also cannot glean from an assessment of misaligned static posture if their alignment improves when they move (Box 5-3).

It is important to assess dynamic alignment in patients before judging and forming conclusions based on static posture. It is important to take the time to assess if they can correct or minimize some of these alignment issues through your cueing. If you see that after several sessions they are doing the best they can with their strategy and still have bony alignment issues without pain, then we can assume that for now this is their ideal posture. Conversely, if the alignment issues remaining are impairing their performance, it may be a signal to refer them to get a structural consultation. Interestingly, poor alignment does not always correlate with or cause pathology. Many famous elite athletes and performers have performed at very high levels with less-than-ideal alignment and never complained of pain or pathology.

When bony alignment issues are apparent, my strategy is to work from center/proximal body parts to the distal extremities. I start by making sure there is good alignment from the pelvis to the spine and thorax, the pelvis to the femur, the femur to the tibia/fibula, the tibia/fibula to the ankle, and the ankle to the foot. If the client can align everything and I find that the client has a true tibial torsion in which the bone itself is externally spiraled, then that becomes their ideal or optimal posture. If they have good alignment proximally, then the rest of the body can align off that even if that means it does not look "correct." It is important not to force the body to look a certain way but rather to facilitate optimal performance within the given structure.

BOX 5-3

I had a patient who was diagnosed with a degenerative joint disease in her knee; her doctors wanted to prepare her for knee surgery. She came walking in with a walker and had severe genu valgum on her right leg. One of the things I find important with an intake is to ask a lot of questions to establish a history of movement, therapy, and overall health. Through this, I found out that she had had both her hips replaced about 6 years before. I asked her the following questions: "Who did your rehabilitation?" and "What kind of exercises do you do?" She replied, "I have never done exercises; I was never prescribed physical therapy, and I was told by my doctor that I can just go back to my normal activities." What stuck out to me is that she had both of her hips done at the same time without ever re-educating the posterior rotators or abductors of either of her hips. Imagine what happens if there is no external rotation or abduction of the hips; the knees collapse in. With a small amount of alignment work, she was able to find close-to-optimal alignment through her knee joint, and based on that single session, I was able to discern that she did not have structural genu valgum at all. It was a genu valgus strategy or the lack of a solid alignment strategy for her lower extremities.

I have seen some movement teachers try to correct from the bottom up. They align the foot and the toes and end up pushing the knees into valgus, sometimes creating more problems in alignment and stress through the knees and hips and the back than there were to begin with. Again, I prefer to work from the center out. Once this is done, any structural malalignment can be accepted, and the client can be taught to modify certain exercises so they can have a positive movement experience without pain or stress. Common misalignments include scoliosis, pelvic torsion, valgus and varus knees, overpronation of the feet, and hallux valgus (bunions). It is important to understand that many people have these variations of bony structures and function fully and without pain, whereas others who have what may seem to be perfect (whatever that means) posture are always injured or in pain.

I have waited until now to discuss foot and ankle mechanics, another of my favorite parts of the body. This might be because of my fascination with dancing and running, 2 activities that are thought to be incredibly tough on feet and often result in foot pathologies. The foot can be divided into 3 parts or 3 axes: the talocrural joint, the medial foot, and the lateral foot (see Figures 4-21 and 4-29 in Chapter 4). When we explore each of these axes of the foot, we can better understand how the foot and ankle are ideally designed to facilitate human gait (Figures 5-10A through 5-10C).

The talocrural joint and how the unique design of the talus and its relationship to the distal tibia and fibular syndesmosis facilitate propulsion through the foot have been discussed previously. When the ankle is in dorsiflexion, the joint becomes more rigid and transfers force into the midfoot and the first and second ray preparing for the toe-off phase of gait.

The medial foot is made up of the talus, navicular, cuneiforms (the medial, intermediate, and lateral), the 3 metatarsals, and the first 3 toes (see Figure 4-21 in Chapter 4). The lateral foot consists of the calcaneus, cuboid, and the lateral 2 metatarsals (4 and 5) and their respective phalanges (see Figure 4-21 in Chapter 4).

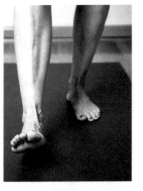 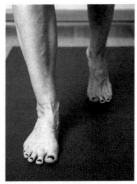 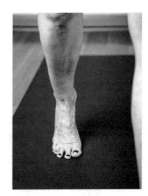

[A]
HEEL STRIKE

[B]
MIDSTANCE

[C]
TOE-OFF

Figure 5-10. The human gait foot contact pattern. (A) Heel strike, (B) midstance, and (C) toe-off.

In the gait cycle starting with the heel strike, the heel comes down with the medial foot supinated and the lateral foot inverted (see Figure 5-10A). Moving from heel strike to midstance or full weight-bearing, the medial foot moves toward pronation and the lateral foot into eversion to absorb ground forces and adapt to uneven surfaces (see Figure 5-10B). Moving from midstance toward toe-off, the body should incline, increasing the dorsiflexion of the ankle and the rigidity of the talocrural joint (see Figure 5-10C). Now here is the exciting part—as the talocrural joint becomes stiff, the lateral foot starts to invert, and the medial foot starts to supinate just enough so that the second metatarsal becomes rigid between the medial and lateral cuneiform, almost like a key, converting the foot to a lever for propulsion (see Figure 4-21 in Chapter 4). Ideally, this propulsion, whether a step or a jump, should convert the elastic energy forward or upward through the second toe, taking advantage of the strong flexor hallucis to finish the toe-off phase of gait.

Figure 5-11 demonstrates normal, supinated, and pronated variations of the foot in midstance. If I see that the footprint splays out in midstance, I know it is overpronated and that the client has possibly lost some of the integrity in the medial foot, or they are lacking proper alignment or bone rhythms in their hips and knees. Again, I always check the hip and knee before I assess the foot and ankle. A great place to facilitate strategic changes for dynamic alignment is on the Pilates reformer. On the reformer, or some other leg press machines, you can set the resistance so the client can perform a high number of repetitions to learn the alignment without getting tired. It is important that the client is being mindful to change their natural pattern toward one that is more ideal. I have observed many clients weight-bearing on their heels in the supine position on the reformer or similar machines and noticed that as they push the carriage out, their feet will change their orientation, even spiraling in different directions. This could be a good indicator of how the ground force might affect the kinetic chain in full vertical weight-bearing.

ARCH TYPE AND FOOT ALIGNMENT

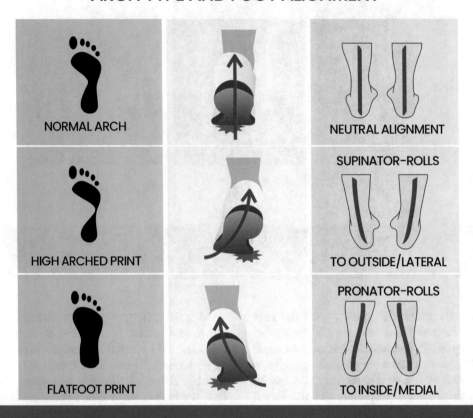

NORMAL ARCH

HIGH ARCHED PRINT

FLATFOOT PRINT

NEUTRAL ALIGNMENT

SUPINATOR-ROLLS

TO OUTSIDE/LATERAL

PRONATOR-ROLLS

TO INSIDE/MEDIAL

Figure 5-11. Three different footprints of the right foot.   (pablofdezr/Shutterstock.com.)

BOX 5-4: GAIT OBSERVATION

Observe your own mechanics as you repeat the midstance, single-leg heel strike, swing, and toe-off phases of gait. Observe what you feel in the medial and lateral foot group of bones, the ankle, the knee, and the hip. If you can, film yourself so you can observe your walking and compare it to what you sense internally. Observe what happens when you change the tempo.

- Midstance
- Single-leg heel strike
- Swing
- Toe-off

MOTOR CONTROL

The first question pertaining to motor control is the following: What does normal movement look like? This is when the anatomical knowledge and the biomechanical knowledge become imperative. The movement practitioner must develop their eye for dynamic alignment and the skill to observe the mover and their ability to maintain optimal congruence of the joints throughout the entire task or activity. Alignment and congruence can be considered more important than strength and flexibility. Becoming familiar with the movement of the joints through their physiological and accessory motion patterns is imperative to becoming a skilled movement practitioner and teacher. In yoga, Pilates, and martial arts, power and mobility are trained simultaneously. Each discipline is mindful of alignment and makes changes to load and tempo throughout the training. Alignment, tempo, and load are crucial in ensuring that the right stresses are being applied to the right tissues in the right time.

Panjabi's model of stability teaches us that there needs to be a balance between noncontractile structures, contractile structures, and the central control of movement.[18,19] This is discussed further in Chapter 6. Once we understand what the normal noncontractile structures look like in the movement model, we can then imagine what the contractile tissues are doing to optimize efficiency in the desired movement task. The myofascial tissues connect to the skeleton, creating elastic and contractile forces on the skeleton and providing the right amount of tension to produce the desired movement outcome. How much is the right amount? This can be confusing sometimes because we do not really know. There are so many muscles involved in every human movement that it would be next to impossible to monitor every muscle by electromyography, especially needle electromyography.

I have found that the best way to facilitate the proper neuromuscular response for a task is by creating the proper alignment, load, and tempo associated with the desired movement pattern. If we can do this and use meaningful cueing, we can communicate with the nervous system. The alternative to this model is trying to teach through muscle contraction cueing (eg, "pull your navel to spine," "squeeze your glutes," "contract your VMO [vastus medialis oblique]," or "lift up your pelvic floor"). Even though all these cues have good intentions, alone they do not contribute to spontaneous and natural movement. If the bones, connective tissue, and fascia are aligned well, then the muscle groups do not have to work nearly as hard as they do in a body that has poor alignment and poor fascial organization. If we find ourselves over-recruiting muscles to move, there is more than likely a problem with alignment, joint congruence, or strategy.

The most common faulty movement patterns in the lower extremity start with a loss of hip control. When the hip cannot control or decelerate internal rotation in midstance, the femur will medially rotate and adduct, which will lead to valgus knees, an everted hindfoot, and a pronated forefoot. A common intervention is to try to correct the alignment from the foot up through orthotics, but if the problem is poor hip organization, the orthotics will only exacerbate the problems in the kinetic chain. Another common faulty movement pattern in the lower kinetic chain is weakness in the hip abductors and external rotators. When this is deficient, you will see the body pitch over the leg to maintain a center of gravity in single-leg weight-bearing. This can be due to many restrictions that need to be assessed. A lack of ankle dorsiflexion is a common reason to turn the hips out to shorten the lever at toe-off. It could also be pain in the knee with midstance, so the client wants to shorten the stride length. Lastly, if the hip is painful or restricted in adduction, flexion, and internal rotation, we may see an altered movement pattern. For those who are not licensed to diagnose, remember that the greatest contributors to faulty movement patterns in the lower extremity typically can fall into poor ankle dorsiflexion and poor hip mechanics. I always check these 2 areas first even if the knee is the painful or dysfunctional joint. Movement teachers can easily incorporate movements designed to improve ankle mobility and good hip alignment, mobility, and control.

The upper extremity is no different in its ability to organize efficiently. As humans, we have many poor postural and movement patterns in the upper extremities (the same as we do in the lower extremities). One way that I look at the efficient or inefficient organization of the upper extremity is by observing the congruence of the humerus with the scapula during movement. If the humeral head is congruent with the glenoid fossa of the scapula, you can observe that the spine of the scapula and the clavicle both point to the center of the humeral head (Figure 5-12; see Figure 4-33 in Chapter 4).

Faulty movement patterns in the upper extremity often involve faulty organization of the scapula with the rib cage. One of the most common is a winging scapula. This is usually caused by a flat thoracic spine and is not really a problem with the scapulae. For the serratus anterior to work efficiently and pull the scapulae into the rib wall, it is necessary that the thoracic spine curve match the curve of the scapula. If the ribs and thoracic spine are too flat, the serratus anterior cannot maintain the congruence of the scapula with the rib cage. Another common faulty movement is partial anterior subluxation of the head of the humerus in relationship to the glenoid fossa and the acromion. There are many reasons for this faulty movement pattern, including being hyperkyphotic, having a posture with rounded shoulders, anterior myofascial restrictions in the pectoral girdle, inhibition of the rotator cuff, and immobility of the scapula through the upper extremity range of motion. Many of these faulty alignment and organization challenges can be attributed to the modern age of sitting, mobile phones, and suburbia. Another

falsehood I have often heard among colleagues defines scapular stability as the ability to hold the scapula in a "neutral" position while moving the humerus. If you want a sure way to wear down the rotator cuff, continue with that theory. The scapula should be constantly adjusting its position to stay in alignment with the humerus. During the assessment of the shoulder girdle, it will become increasingly obvious from a motor control standpoint that if the thoracic spine and rib cage are immobile, the scapula is unable to maintain congruence through the entire range of the upper extremity. The scapula can move in protraction and retraction, elevation and depression, and upward and downward rotation; however, it is not able to move into extension or flexion or axial rotation. These movements of the scapula are dependent on thoracic spine mobility. A good example of this is the tennis serve or the freestyle swim stroke. If the thoracic spine is

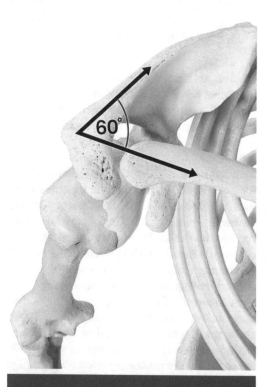

Figure 5-12. A superior view of shoulder alignment.
(SciePro/Shutterstock.com.)

BOX 5-5: THE PERFECT PUSH-UP

Start with a partial weight-bearing experience with the hands on the mat.

First, while in a quadruped position, observe the beginning position of your hand and wrist. You can begin by attempting to press straight fingers into the floor (see Figure 5-9); at the same time, you want to try to extend your wrist. This will spontaneously create the manibandha or cocontraction of the wrist; this will also prevent hyperextension of the elbow.

Second, we want to connect the lower trunk to the upper trunk. Start by lifting the sternum up toward the ceiling as if your back was a sail from a sailboat that just caught wind. Be mindful to keep length in your spine and avoid shoulder protraction. With the hands still in their manibandha position, lift the knees off the ground 1 inch and hover. Repeat this multiple times until you can feel the connection between the head, thoracic cage, and pelvis. I call this the *beast position*, which is used in Animal Flow.

Third, in the quadruped position, walk your hands out until the body is in a kneeling plank position. Bring your attention to the connected feeling of the trunk and the manibandha of the wrist and hand. Now allow the elbows to glide back as you allow the shoulders to spin in their sockets forward. Note that the scapula will move and this is normal. Repeat a half-kneeling push-up in kneeling plank multiple times until you are comfortable with the bone rhythm of the elbow and shoulder; the key word is "allowing" the joints to do their job of hinging, spinning, and gliding.

Fourth, put it all together. Start in your third position, and lift the knees and sternum at the same time, making that elastic connection between the pelvis and trunk. Press your ribs and thighs up as you press the pelvis forward until you are in a long diagonal line. Because you are in a full push-up plank position now, you are ready for half-range push-ups. Allow the elbows to bend back and the shoulders to spin forward. Repeat multiple times. As you feel more comfortable with the plank position and the bone rhythms of the upper extremity, challenge yourself to perform three-quarter push-ups and then full push-ups. Keep bringing your attention back to manibandha and the sternum/thigh lift when you are feeling like you are collapsing.

not able to move into extension and rotation, then the glenohumeral joint will take up the excessive movement and force in the form of subluxation or shear forces on the labrum. My patients tell me when they are diagnosed with a rotator cuff injury that their physician says "80% of adults over the age of 50 years who are active will end up with rotator cuff injuries." This is a cop-out. What they should be saying is that if we intend to age actively (eg, playing tennis or golf; running; swimming; cycling; hiking; climbing; playing volleyball,

basketball, or baseball), we should make sure we keep our thoracic spine supple, especially in extension and rotation.

Another common alignment challenge in the upper extremity is hyperextension of the elbows. Most humans are not used to bearing weight through their upper extremities unless they practice certain martial arts; do push-ups and calisthenics; or are gymnasts, modern dancers, pole-vaulters, or other athletes who use their upper extremities in a closed kinetic chain. Mike Fitch, Ido Portal, and many others have brought high-level movement exploration into focus. I would check out their work if you have a chance. Because of the unfamiliarity, when people bear weight in their arms, they do not know how to suspend themselves to find balance between the skeleton and the myofascial system. This leads to load at the path of least resistance (ie, the elbows). Hyperextended elbows are often accompanied by a hyperextended wrist and winging scapula, which move the disfunction up the chain and into the trunk. The idea of the cocontraction in the wrist, which was discussed previously in this chapter, can help with this faulty movement pattern. Hopefully, as movement teachers, we will be sticklers about upper extremity alignment.

Rather than focusing on faulty movement patterns, let us focus on how to move more efficiently. How do we facilitate accurate alignment? This is necessary for efficient transfer of forces between these bones moving through space. When we understand the relationship of the kinetic chain and arthrokinematics, it is easier for us to understand how body weight will transfer through space. This does not mean that we are always vertical. I have a dance background, and a lot of movement that I did was lying on my back, rolling around, doing gymnastics, and flipping through the air.

It becomes essential to understand the relationships between the anatomy and the forces applied to the anatomical structures. The orientation with gravity is not nearly as important as the ability to maintain proper dynamic alignment and joint congruence. This allows for a more spontaneous and balanced reaction when our joints are aligned properly. Congruent joints also increase the dynamic stability of a joint. When we have congruence, we feel that we can accelerate faster, adapt quicker to abnormal forces, and enhance performance. Therefore, many elite athletes take Pilates, yoga, Feldenkrais Method, and Gyrotonic Expansion System classes. Cirque du Soleil has a staff of physical therapists, Pilates and yoga instructors, and nutritionists

on call for its performers because they believe in the concept of dynamic alignment to prevent injuries and maximize performance. They are convinced that it saves them money and time by keeping their performers healthy. It also improves the quality of their performance. Not just elite performers need to enhance their alignment; everyone needs to improve alignment, including grandparents so they can pick up their grandchildren without being afraid of hurting their back or knees (Box 5-6).

BIOENERGETICS

In the Hawaiian Islands, there was an ancient spiritual belief called *Huna*. Maybe you have heard of the great kahuna. The kahuna was the shaman in the Polynesian islands' spiritual belief Huna. The kahuna's job was to align the subconscious spirit with the conscious spirit. In the Hawaiian Islands, they believe that when the conscious and subconscious are aligned, the individual is

BOX 5-6

When my children were young, we had a neighbor who was 95 years old. Her name was Gladys. She would get on the ground with our children and play with them. She also told us how her mother and grandmother had a horrible dowager's hump; she did not want to have one, so she would stand up next to the wall every day to make sure she had good posture. I will never forget watching her get up and down off the ground without using her hands. Thank you, Gladys, for that life lesson. It just goes to show that we are what we practice.

aligned with the "Great Spirit" (ie, the universe). It was common that the kahunas could be male or female, and they helped the people transition through stages of spiritual growth and physical, emotional, mental, and spiritual fulfillment.[20]

As previously mentioned, when people are aligned physically, mentally, and spiritually, the systems of the body seem to function better. When our systems function better, the mind is clearer, we tend to think better, and we tend to perform better at work. We tend to be happier and kinder. We tend to see things in the world as being more beautiful. Alignment is everything.

We know that all our energy passes through the areas going up into our head and our shoulders. The meridians of acupuncture pass through our shoulders. These are called the *mu points*. Whether the loss of posture came first and we started having congestion in these mu points, or we had some problems with our lung or gallbladder and some of those meridians before and lost our posture, is not as important as the restoration of normal function and energetic flow through all the meridians. These are all important aspects of improving the quality of our health. A visit to the acupuncturist can significantly open the flow of chi through the nociceptive stimuli in different meridians of the body. The needle placement is based on a 5000-year-old system that balances the many systems in the body. When poor posture compromises these meridians, it must restrict the energetic flow through the body and the associated organs.

Good posture makes for healthy moving, healthy organs, and healthy energy flow and builds up our immune system; it can even improve the way we think or the way we perceive ourselves. It is amazing how important our self-efficacy and our self-esteem can be built by something as simple as posture.

OPEN-ENDED QUESTIONS

1 Explain in your own words how "alignment" can be used to define the congruence of joints and bones, as well as congruence between perception and reality. How does one's perception of their body in space relate to actual structural alignment?

2 How can poor posture of the axial skeleton affect mobility and control?

3 A sagittal line rising vertically from the second toe is likely to intersect which joints and bony landmarks? Explain how this vertical alignment of the lower extremity into the trunk can influence center of gravity.

4 Make a list of comparisons between the hip and the glenohumeral joint for congruency, arthrokinematics, osteokinematics, planes of movement, muscle attachments, cartilage, degrees of freedom, capsule, stability, etc.

5 Make a list of comparisons between the knee and the elbow joint, congruency, arthrokinematics, osteokinematics, planes of movement, muscle attachments, cartilage, degrees of freedom, capsule, stability, etc.

6 Make a list of comparisons between the distal leg and forearm joint, congruency, arthrokinematics, osteokinematics, planes of movement, muscle attachments, cartilage, degrees of freedom, capsule, stability, etc.

OPEN-ENDED QUESTIONS

7 Describe what might be the disadvantages of using static vs dynamic alignment to assess functional movements. Give an example of when you have made an assessment error in relying on static alignment assessment. What did you notice?

8 Give examples of common static malalignments that are often catastrophized. What can happen to the client's self-belief if less important static malalignments are focused on?

9 Explain the gait cycle from heel strike to toe-off. What is proper dynamic alignment at each phase of the gait cycle: midstance, single-leg heel strike, swing, and toe-off? What is the purpose in normal gait of a more rigid toe-off vs a more relaxed midfoot?

10 Give an example of how poor hip internal rotation deceleration can affect the entire lower extremity. What is the hip unable to control?

11 What is an example of an intervention strategy where the hallux valgus is excessive and painful, and you are charged to treat the big toe alignment? Give both an example of working with the foot up and one working from the hip down. Which do you feel will be more effective and why?

12 Rotator cuff impingement is a common diagnosis for active older adults. Give a hypothesis of what might lead to subacromial impingements of the rotator cuff. Where else could you focus the mobility and alignment training to relieve the stress under the acromion with overhead activity?

13 Explain how exercises that incorporate mindfulness and awareness may result in alignment of mind and body. Journal how awareness exercises have influenced your well-being. How can you share this experience with your clients?

REFERENCES

1. Franklin EN. *Conditioning for Dance*. Human Kinetics; 2004.
2. Bogduk N, Twomey LT. *Clinical Anatomy of the Lumbar Spine*. Churchill Livingstone; 1987.
3. Bordoni B, Lintonbon D, Morabito B. Meaning of the solid and liquid fascia to reconsider the model of biotensegrity. *Cureus*. 2018;10(7):e2922.
4. Bordoni B, Simonelli M. The awareness of the fascial system. *Cureus*. 2018;10(10):e3397.
5. Pilates JH, Robbins J, Van Heuit-Robbins L. *Pilates Evolution: The 21st Century*. Presentation Dynamics; 2012.
6. Ray MB. Cutting a fine figure. *Reader's Digest*. October 29, 1934.
7. Kulkarni V, Chandy M, Babu K. Quantitative study of muscle spindles in suboccipital muscles of human foetuses. *Neurol India*. 2001;49(4):355-359.
8. Cullen KE, Brooks JX, Sadeghi SG. How actions alter sensory processing. *Ann N Y Acad Sci*. 2009;1164(1):29-36.
9. Earls J. *Born to Walk: Myofascial Efficiency and the Body in Movement*. North Atlantic Books; 2014.
10. Earls J, Myers TW. *Fascial Release for Structural Balance*. North Atlantic Books; 2010.
11. Myers TW. *Anatomy Trains: Myofascial Meridians for Manual and Movement Therapists*. 3rd ed. Elsevier; 2014.

12. Harrison DE, Cailliet R, Harrison DD, Janik TJ. How do anterior/posterior translations of the thoracic cage affect the sagittal lumbar spine, pelvic tilt, and thoracic kyphosis? *Eur Spine J*. 2002;11(3):287-293.

13. Harrison DE, Colloca CJ, Harrison DD, Janik TJ, Haas JW, Keller TS. Anterior thoracic posture increases thoracolumbar disc loading. *Eur Spine J*. 2005;14(3):234-242.

14. Harrison DE, Janik TJ, Cailliet R, et al. Upright static pelvic posture as rotations and translations in 3-dimensional from three 2-dimensional digital images: validation of a computerized analysis. *J Manipulative Physiol Ther*. 2008;31(2):137-145.

15. Harrison DE, Jones EW, Janik TJ, Harrison DD. Evaluation of axial and flexural stresses in the vertebral body cortex and trabecular bone in lordosis and two sagittal cervical translation configurations with an elliptical shell model. *J Manipulative Physiol Ther*. 2002;25(6):391-401.

16. Calais-Germain B. *Anatomy of Movement*. Eastland Press; 2007.

17. Borg-Olivier S. *Applied Anatomy & Physiology of Yoga*. Warisanoffset.com; 2006.

18. Panjabi MM. The stabilizing system of the spine. Part II. Neutral zone and instability hypothesis. *J Spinal Disord*. 1992;5(4):390-396; discussion 397.

19. Panjabi MM. The stabilizing system of the spine. Part I. Function, dysfunction, adaptation, and enhancement. *J Spinal Disord*. 1992;5(4):383-389; discussion 397.

20. What is Huna. ancientHuna.com. 2005. http://www.ancienthuna.com/what_is_huna.htm

CONTROL

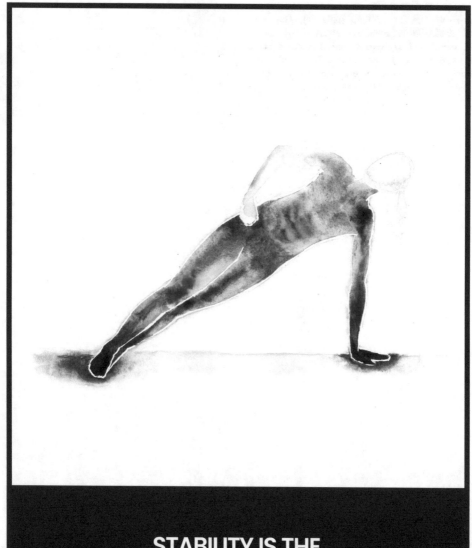

**STABILITY IS THE
CONTROL OF MOBILITY.**

CHAPTER 6

CHAPTER OBJECTIVES

1 Comprehend the movement professional's definition of stability as control of mobility and resilience to external perturbations.

2 Describe the progression of learning novel movement from one of volitional over-recruitment to one of spontaneous subconscious adjustments to load.

3 Comprehend how to create a spontaneous response by using exercises that demand proper neuromuscular adaptation.

4 Understand the applications of the different kinetic chains that mimic functional activities, as well as those that can be used to initiate graded loading and be progressed into a normal orientation to gravity and movement forces. This includes open chain, closed chain, and pseudo-closed chain kinetics.

5 Understand and identify how and when the body compensates after injury resulting in local muscle inhibition and global muscle excitation.

6 Familiarize self with current vernacular of control, including core control, neutral zone, stability, intra-abdominal pressure (IAP), proprioception, stiffness, and mobility. (Readers will express how they are similar and different in movement science and how it can be applied.)

KEY TERMS

- Anticipated load
- Closed kinetic
- Compensatory patterns
- Control
- Deep/local muscles
- Endurance
- Force couples
- Genetic predispositions
- Global muscles
- Graded load
- Gravity
- Habitual patterns
- Hydraulic amplifier
- Intra-abdominal pressure
- Kinetic chains
- Load
- Neutral spine
- Neutral zone
- Open kinetic
- Pain excitation
- Pain inhibition
- Pseudo-closed kinetic
- Repetitions
- Spontaneous organization
- Stability
- Synergistic organization
- Valsalva technique

Control has a direct relationship with mobility. When mobility is present in a joint complex, such as the lumbopelvic region or the shoulder girdle, it becomes necessary that there is a balance between neuromuscular control, stability of the noncontractile structures, and the proper tone and timing of the contractile tissues surrounding the joints. This balance or integrated control is necessary to achieve efficient and spontaneous movement. In this chapter, control and load as they pertain to human movement are discussed.

- 125 -

Anderson BD.
Principles of Movement (pp 124-148).
© 2024 Taylor & Francis Group.

Control is often used synonymously in movement science with stability. However, in medicine and surgery, the word stability is often synonymous with rigidity or fixation (ie, the lumbar spine is stable after the fusion). This use of the word "stable" does not apply in the teaching of this book and should not be confused with the control of mobility or the attempt to volitionally brace a part of the body; rather, stability should be about facilitating the appropriate amount of stiffness around motion segments and joints in the body per the anticipated load.

STABILITY IS THE CONTROL OF MOBILITY.

Joseph Pilates' original concepts of whole body movement focused on the ability for us to move naturally and spontaneously and participate in our many daily activities with zest and pleasure.[1] To have natural and spontaneous movement, motor control needs to be spontaneous as it reacts to conscious and subconscious movement tasks and the external and internal loads that affect the body's organization to accomplish the desired tasks.

Load can manifest in external forces influencing the human body, including gravity, momentum, repetitions, tempo, and endurance, and can also manifest in the form of internal forces, such as tensile forces. According to Schleip et al,[2] we need to think of our bodies in relationship to posture and movement having a dominance in tensional load rather than compressive load. In the tensegrity model, the tensional elements are all connected with one another in a global tension-transmitting network.[3] This is an exciting new way of looking at movement driven by a higher quality of tensegrity-like qualities or elasticity in the movement.[2] This concept of the skeleton being sprung by the myofascial tissues over the axial skeleton in its optimal axial alignment results in the 3-dimensional organization of the torso moving with more desirable efficiency and elasticity. When the bones are in a tensional state through proper structural alignment, the healthy body will be springy and efficient and minimize structural deformation.

CONTROL OF THE TRUNK AND PELVIS

The transverse abdominis (TA), multifidus, and pelvic floor muscles have received a lot of attention over the past 30 years as being primary local stabilizers of the lumbopelvic region.[4-11] These local stabilizers typically work subconsciously and in a subthreshold state, which means we often will not be aware of them while they are working. Another important concept is how these muscles work synergistically. The complexity of how all our muscles work together in harmony and balance can be difficult to comprehend. I refer to it as an orchestra in which many instruments are playing together to create beautiful music. Some muscles create local stiffness and are playing pianissimo, some create acceleration, or in music a crescendo, some create deceleration or a decrescendo, and some muscles approximate a bone closer together to create congruence of the joint, like percussion instruments that keep the rhythm and alignment of the other instruments in the orchestra. The entire neuromuscular system is attempting to work harmoniously to facilitate spontaneous movement. This fills me with awe and appreciation for the magnificence of our bodies.

It helps to understand which muscles are responsible for stabilization/control and which are responsible for movement (ie, acceleration/deceleration). Knowledge pertaining to the nature of local and global muscles and their actions can only edify our observation skills of movement efficiency and movement strategy. We can trust that the neuromuscular system will respond appropriately based on the body's alignment and anticipated load to match the desired task. What I mean by this is that sometimes we get in our own way by attempting to contract muscles volitionally instead of naturally. I remember early on in my career practicing and trying to isolate the contraction of muscles that we knew were important muscles, such as the TA or the pubococcygeus, but we did not know how to facilitate the contraction.

What should the timing be or how much contraction is enough? We also did not know how
they should work with actual trunk movement
because we could not perform needle electromyography while the spine was moving. We
would facilitate a conscious contraction of the
TA and still not be able to convert it to a spontaneous one, as demonstrated in the study
by Hodges and Richardson[8] in 1996. We later
found out that this was not an effective way
to facilitate efficient movement or contraction
of these local stabilizers. However, when we
shifted our focus from muscle contraction to
alignment and load, we were able to facilitate
spontaneous activation of the TA simply by
aligning the rib cage, pelvis, and spine axially and applying a sufficient load to the axial
skeleton.

ESSENTIAL SCIENCES
ANATOMY

Let us revisit the muscles of the trunk (see
Figure 3-7B in Chapter 3). The rectus abdominis is the anterior pillar of the abdominal
wall. Its fibers run vertically. It is segmented
by fascial connections, and its primary purpose is to accelerate or decelerate flexion and
extension of the spine.[2,12-14] When this muscle
contracts, it shortens and pulls the lower rib
cage and sternum down toward the pubis or
the pubis up toward the sternum. If nothing
else is synergistically happening from neuromuscular organization in the trunk, the result
will simply be approximation of the anterior
space of the trunk. When it contracts, the rectus abdominis shortens the anterior pillar of
the body.

The oblique abdominal muscles are oriented perpendicular to each other and in diagonals with the body. It was discussed briefly
in Chapter 5 that the external oblique and
the external intercostal muscles run in the
same direction as if I were placing my hands
into my pockets. It is a 45-degree angle to the
rectus abdominis. The internal obliques are

perpendicular (90 degrees) to the external
obliques, and again, at a 45-degree angle into
the rectus abdominis. We have this beautiful
cross on the side of our abdominal wall that
connects to the fascia of the rectus abdominis
or the anterior pillar. The internal abdominal
oblique muscles also connect posteriorly to the
thoracolumbar fascia. The external abdominal
oblique muscles connect to the rib cage anteriorly, and together the obliques are designed to
balance the position of the thorax over the pelvis. If I over-recruit any of these muscles, I will
lose the alignment/balance. These abdominal
muscles should be working synergistically and
subconsciously to maintain the relationship of
the rib cage to the pelvis and respond directly
to the spinal movement and gravity or other
external loads on the spine, not excluding the
quadratus lumborum and other muscles in
the back of the trunk doing the same. This is
discussed in more depth later in this section.

The fibers of the TA run horizontally or
90 degrees in relation to the pillar of the rectus abdominis (see Figure 3-7B in Chapter 3).
These muscle fibers do not have a direction of
movement on the body like the obliques or the
rectus abdominis. They approximate the anterior, lateral, and posterior walls of the trunk
toward the central axis. It is a unique property that the TA muscle provides, hence all the
attention in the core control literature. It is a
preparatory muscle for the control of movement and the anticipation of load. It is thought
that the TA and its synergies with other local
stabilizers are responsible for much of the stiffness in the spine referred to in the yoga world
as *mula bandha*.[15,16] The TA creates the proper
amount of stiffness to the spine based on the
anticipated load or experience.

The TA will fire subconsciously and subthreshold in anticipation of movement. It does
not matter if you are moving your arms or
legs, or bending or lifting something, the TA
will create enough stiffness and IAP for efficient and fluid movement.[8] If we look at the
horizontal slice of the rectus abdominis and the
abdominal wall in Figure 6-1, we see something
very interesting, especially in the middle slice.

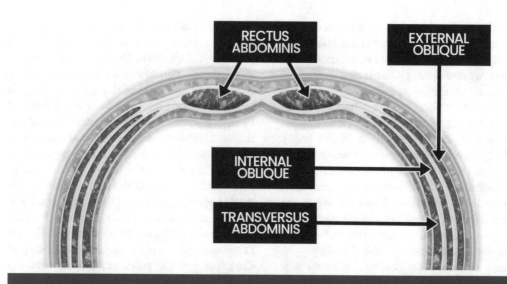

Figure 6-1. A cross section of the abdominal wall.

Observe the fascial sheath that surrounds the rectus abdominis. The rectus abdominis sheath is made up of the fascial layers/tendons of the other abdominal muscles. If we were to go from superficial to deep, the most superficial muscle would be the external oblique. The external oblique runs in a 45-degree angle as if the hands are going in the pockets. Those fibers make up the anterior wall of the rectus abdominis sheath. The internal oblique that runs 90 degrees perpendicular to the external oblique comes in and split its fibers. Half of them go around the front of the rectus abdominis sheath, and the other half go around the posterior, creating an envelope around the muscle of the rectus abdominis, like a jelly-filled donut.

The TA approaches horizontally underneath the internal oblique and makes up the fascial layer deep to the rectus abdominis. With this view, one can see how the rectus belly is enveloped by the fascia coming in from these 3 different angles. Imagine moving your body through space or swinging a golf club or a tennis racket. These muscles might fire at different times to create just enough stiffness in anticipation of the load to keep us on that central axis and optimize the movement of our spine in the rotation of a tennis swing, the throwing of

a ball, or the kicking of a soccer ball (Figures 6-2A and 6-2B). We can also imagine the myofascial connectivity creating an efficient elasticity to the movement across the torso. In any of these activities, these muscles work synergistically and harmoniously in a very experienced mover. In someone who has been injured, we see just the opposite. We see an inhibition of these deep local stabilizers resulting in faulty compensation of these muscles because of pain, fear, or loss of structural stability.

The TA has another unique property. As previously mentioned, the TA wraps all the way around the body and connects to the posterior lumbar fascia or the thoracolumbar fascia. It draws on the rectus sheath and the thoracolumbar fascia. The thoracolumbar fascial sheath is filled with the erector spinae and multifidus muscles. Notice on the ultrasound pictures in Figures 6-3A and 6-3B that you can see the curve of the TA coming around the body; it thickens as it contracts to draw the abdominal wall in (see Figure 6-3B).

Just like the anterior wall, there is a vertical pillar on the back, which is called the *erector spinae* (see Figure 4-10 in Chapter 4). The erector spinae is made up of several muscles

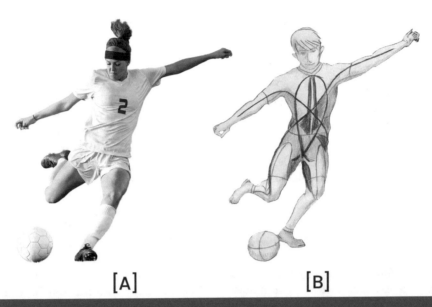

Figure 6-2. (A) A soccer player. (B) Myofascial depiction of the same soccer player.

(JoeSAPhotos/Shutterstock.com.)
(Illustrated by Kelly Anderson.)

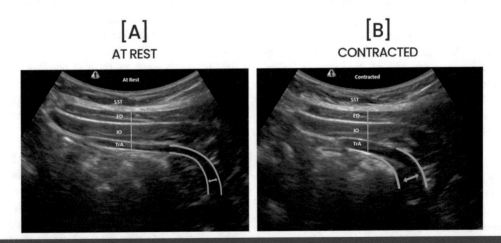

[A] AT REST

[B] CONTRACTED

Figure 6-3. Ultrasound images of the TA (A) at rest and (B) contracted.

that run vertical in the body and connect onto the spine process, the transverse process, or the ribs directly. They all originate from the pelvic rim or the lumbar spine. These muscles run vertical, just like the rectus abdominis, and have an action arm of extension. When these muscles contract, they shorten the space and facilitate extension or compression in the low back, almost like a guide wire on an antenna tower on a building.[10] Again, we need that axial length to come from those other muscles (ie, the TA, oblique, multifidus, and pelvic floor muscles) to be able to have efficient extension or flexion.[8] The large muscle of the latissimus dorsi (see Figure 4-38 in Chapter 4) comes down from the arm and connects the upper extremity into the thoracolumbar fascia. This is a diagonal muscle that acts like the obliques do in the front. It provides a similar tension angle to the external obliques, angling into the thoracolumbar fascia in the back and creating reciprocal tensile forces posteriorly.

Deep inside the thoracolumbar fascia are the deep muscles of the back, including the multifidus and interosseous muscles. These muscles do not really have movement properties as far as direction of movement, but they create stiffness in multiple planes. They create the appropriate amount of control or stability around the spine based on the anticipated load related to the activity. The other unique quality about the multifidus muscle is that it contains more than 6 times the average number of muscle spindle fibers. These are your proprioceptive fibers (or information fibers of where your spine is in space). When these muscles are healthy, they are also hypertrophied inside of that thoracolumbar fascial envelope. They can create a stiffness physiologically.[10] This method of stiffening the local muscles around the lumbar spine can be referred to as the *guide wire model of stability*. Hypertrophy of the muscles inside of the fascial envelope create a stiffening and stabilizing effect for large loads, such as powerlifting, in which the trunk requires additional stiffness to prevent migration or shear force from doing harm to the spine tissues. The fascial slings can also create significant tension and control with little force, resulting in significant control and stability of its underlying structures, including the anterior abdominal wall and the rectus abdominis sheath.[2,12-14]

The psoas major is another important muscle that has multiple roles. The superior medial fibers act like local stabilizers, creating lateral stiffness of the spinal segments where the long fibers of the psoas can act like a global muscle aiding with hip flexion. The psoas major ascends and has a relationship with the lumbar and inferior thoracic spine. It ascends past the lumbar spine and has insertions up through the diaphragm into the lower thoracic spine in the anterior body or the anterior-lateral body of the vertebra (see Figure 4-12 in

Chapter 4). This is very important regarding the connectivity and integration between the lower extremities and their effect on axial alignment and stability of the torso.

If an individual is standing in an anterior pelvic tilt, the pull of the psoas major muscle is behind the central axial line and can create a shear force on the lumbar spine. Contrarily, when the spine is in a relatively neutral or slightly flexed posture, the psoas has a mechanical advantage because of the stiffness surrounding the lumbar and lower thoracic spinal segments at the origin of the muscle. The local fibers of the psoas in this region provide support and stiffness surrounding the vertebrae to increase the efficiency of hip flexion, especially with the long lever movement of the lower extremity against gravity.

It is best to trust that these muscles, when the skeleton has aligned correctly, will work efficiently based on the load, whether it be gravity, tempo, or endurance. This results in increased power in our kicking, running, and jumping. It is quite common for patients with lumbar pathology to have overactive psoas major and quadratus lumborum muscles and inhibited local stabilizers (eg, the TA and multifidus), resulting in unwanted shear force with standing activities.

Another muscle group that is part of the organization of the hydraulic amplifier is the pelvic floor muscles. The pubococcygeus muscle has fascial connections to other muscles, including the deep rotator muscles of the hip, such as the obturator internus and externus, the gemelli muscles, and the piriformis that originates from the anterior ala of the sacrum. The iliacus muscle originates on the anterior crest of the iliac, whereas the iliopsoas tendon inserts on the lesser trochanter located on the medial side of the femur. All these have a very intricate relationship to maintain the body in an upright and vertical position. It is a miracle that we can stand and locomote so easily. Faulty control of the pelvic and hip musculature, either working too much or too little, can lead to other types of compensations that can cause impairments, complications, or secondary pathologies. I want to emphasize that the muscles of the pelvic sling are part of the intra-abdominal cylinder referred to as the *hydraulic amplifier* by Norris[11] (see Figure 3-5 in Chapter 3) that helps control the IAP. If we have too much constriction or too much contraction in our abdominal wall and we attempt to hold our abdominal wall in all the time, the core can become ineffective. This can be observed in overzealous Pilates and exercise teachers who over-recruit their abdominal wall so much that the internal abdominal oblique muscles become immobile and may result in a contracture of the anterior abdominal wall. It no longer allows the wall to expand; therefore, the diaphragm does not descend, and the pelvic floor potentially loses its elastic nature and spontaneous reaction to load. This may manifest as a hypertonic or hypotonic pelvic floor musculature. When the pelvic floor loses its elasticity and spontaneity, it may lead to problems such as incontinence or other pelvic floor dysfunctions. Note the ultrasound images in Figures 6-4A and 6-4B of pelvic floors that are contracting but descending because of over-recruitment of the abdominal wall compared with the normal ascending and descending that occurs with breath or spontaneous movement. As our knowledge of the effect that

load and control have on the trunk grows, it is necessary to study how the lower extremity reacts to load and integrates with the trunk. We will also look at the kinetic chains and see the effect they have on whole body movement.

APPLICATION
LOAD OF THE EXTREMITIES THROUGH THE KINETIC CHAINS

Biomechanics and arthrokinematics are directly related to the kinetic chains acting on and through the extremities to improve or challenge the organization of the body's movement. The kinetic chain allows us to understand properties of movement and can be used to enhance the movement experience for the client and match the level of the client's movement consciousness with the appropriate load. Kinetic chains are divided into 3 categories. In this book, they are referred to as *closed kinetic chain*, *open kinetic chain*, and *pseudo-closed kinetic chain*. In movement re-education, we use all 3 of these, some more than others. The Pilates method has unique attributes in

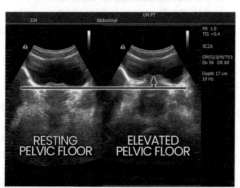
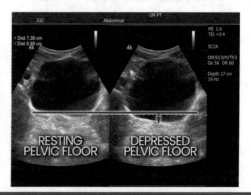

Figure 6-4. Real-time ultrasound images of the pelvic floor. (A) Normal elevation of the pelvic floor. (B) Abnormal depression of the pelvic floor.

its use of assistance and gravity elimination. We have learned a great deal from Pilates and how it can use all 3 categories of kinetic chain activity to restore movement and enhance performance.

Closed chain kinetics is when the distal aspect of the extremity, usually the hand or foot, is fixed against a stable surface. The proximal body part then moves on top of the fixed distal body part. For example, when performing a squat standing on the floor, the feet are on the floor (the distal body part on a fixed surface) and the upper leg torso (the proximal part) moves on top of the fixed foot bearing weight on the floor. The knees and hips are bending as you squat. The proximal (closest to the trunk) part is moving on the distal. A push-up is the same in the upper body. The hand is fixed on the floor, and the wrist, elbow, shoulder, and scapula are where movement occurs.

If we think about a bench press, the movement is the same as a push-up, but the hands are no longer against a nonmoving surface. This is called an open chain exercise. Open chain kinetics make up most of our daily tasks and can be defined as the distal aspect of the limb moving on the proximal part of the body (eg, throwing or kicking a ball). Why are each of these kinetic chains important to movement science?

In rehabilitation science, we often find ourselves with patients who have lost control of a limb or joint after an injury or accident. If you have ever sprained your ankle, you might have noticed that once it heals, it is hard to balance, and sometimes it just does not feel the same. This often has to do with proprioception. It is known that a closed chain load in a joint stimulates a much higher percentage of mechanoreceptors and other proprioceptive fibers. This is extremely important early on to establish the awareness of the limb, or more particularly, the joint. You will see this when someone has suffered a neurologic accident such as a stroke and has neglect or hemiparesis. The therapist will use compression and

load on the affected limb in a closed kinetic chain environment. This mechanically stimulates the receptors. Because most human tasks are open chain, we must progress the movement toward open chain activities. The goal of rehabilitation is to restore open chain activity/function. The good news is that we have one more kinetic chain to aid in the transition from closed to open kinetic chain tasks.

The third kinetic chain is one we made up for descriptive purposes; it is called the *pseudo-closed chain* or *pseudo-open chain*. It is neither fully closed nor open. For example, when riding a bicycle, your feet are on the pedals, and even though it is the distal part of the lower extremity that is fixed on the pedals, the pedals are not fixed; hence, it does not meet the definition of a true closed kinetic chain or open chain setting. Therefore, we came up with the term *pseudo-closed chain*. The distal extremity is on a fixed arc of movement, and the foot in this case is getting some support or pushback from the pedal. For example, in Pilates, when we move the tower bar on the trapeze table, it moves on a fixed arc (Figure 6-5). The fixed arc guides the extremity through space in a controlled path. If I had an injury and I did not know how to perform an open chain movement with my arm after shoulder surgery, I could use a pseudo-closed movement to assist in learning how to achieve the desired movement. There will be more feedback and more proprioception with a closed or pseudo-closed chain movement than with an open chain movement. Pilates provides many ways to transition from a closed chain movement through a pseudo-closed chain movement and eventually into an open chain movement. Following are some examples on Pilates equipment.

Footwork on a Pilates reformer is performed with the feet on the foot bar and springs attached below; this Pilates exercise is a clear example of a closed kinetic chain activity. The feet are fixed on a bar that is not moving. As the individual presses into the bar, the body moves in a similar relationship to the feet as in a vertical squat (Figure 6-6).

A pseudo-closed chain activity can be a natural progression to prepare the body to go up and down stairs. The Pilates chair has a bar with springs attached to an anchor. The foot bar moves through a fixed arc of space. As seen in Figure 6-7, as the patient moves her leg, it is resembling normal movement patterning. In this example, the springs are assisting hip and knee flexion similar to the open phase of gait or climbing stairs. Once the client has learned to move correctly with assistance, the progression is to perform this movement without assistance and without guidance, hence open chain kinetics. We use this all the time in Pilates rehabilitation and postrehabilitation. It is important that we can explain what we do to our colleagues, physical therapists and doctors, athletic trainers, and health care professionals. We should also be able to explain this to our clients so they gain the physical and mental confidence to progress and heal.

As mentioned previously, a pseudo-closed chain activity provides a transition from a closed chain to an open chain activity. There is little to no research supporting the biomechanics of a pseudo-closed chain activity, but clinically it can make a lot of sense in the progression from a closed chain to an open chain activity. Clinically speaking, we find that pseudo-closed chain kinematics does facilitate a more effective transition to an open chain or functional movement activity.

Last is the progression into open chain movements, such as walking, marching, swinging the arms, reaching, jumping, and stepping up and down steps. These movements represent the extremities moving through space without external guidance or assistance.

The same rules of the kinetic chains apply to the upper extremities; almost all upper extremity activities involving daily living are open chain. As mentioned earlier, closed chain activities facilitate a cocontraction around the involved joints, which stimulates the mechanoreceptors in the muscles (muscle spindle fibers), as well as the mechanoreceptors in the ligaments around the joint, the Golgi tendon organs of the tendons, and the Golgi organs of

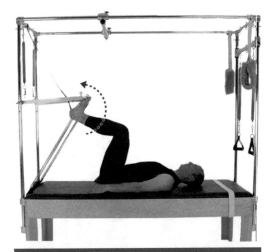

Figure 6-5. Footwork on the trapeze table.

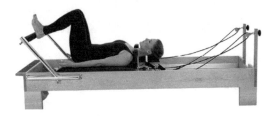

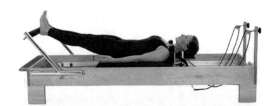

Figure 6-6. Footwork on the reformer.

the fascia. Closed chain movement and loading increase the communication feed mechanism into part of the reticular formation in the brain, which helps with the coordination of the movement, and more importantly, enhanced awareness of our body in space. As mentioned previously, we use closed chain loading with neurologic disorders, such as strokes, multiple sclerosis, head trauma, and spinal cord lesions.

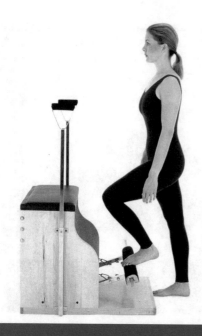

Figure 6-7. A standing leg pump on the chair.

Open chain movement requires practice and repetition to improve awareness and restore function. To increase one's awareness of a feed-forward activity (eg, throwing a ball), it requires external and internal feedback to know if the task was executed correctly. In the example of throwing a ball, the feedback would determine if the ball went where the thrower wanted it to go. If not, the thrower makes small adjustments to refine the movement for next time. It is like a baby learning to eat. They start off with more food on their faces than in their mouths, but with practice, they can finally put the food in their mouths quite well. Another source of feedback that greatly influences the success of feeding is a full tummy (Box 6-1).

MOTOR CONTROL

As previously discussed, control and responsiveness are highly dependent on our movement experiences. Collective motor learning, habituations to behaviors, beliefs

about our abilities to move or not, injury history, and much more influence our response to load. The nervous system has various levels of control, including spinal cord reflexes, lower brain anticipatory responses, and volitional movements. Some are repetitive, and some are unique. This leads us into the need to better understand motor learning and motor control as they pertain to load and spontaneous control of our movement.

SYNERGISTIC AND SPONTANEOUS ORGANIZATION

Let us discuss the concept of the hydraulic amplifier to determine how it pertains to the management of load. The organization of these contractile and noncontractile structures surrounding the axial skeleton can significantly improve axial length. Remember that the hydraulic amplifier is made of the diaphragm from above, the pelvic floor from below, the abdominal muscles around the front, the back muscle in the back, and the TA that connects anterior and posterior with a horizontal orientation (see Figure 3-5). These muscles work synergistically, controlling the IAP. When we think of drawing the structure closer toward the central axis, we are going to feel the posture lengthen. This is different than merely trying to increase the IAP. The strongest IAP can be achieved by integrating the trunk wall, bearing down, and either controlling the airflow or stopping it altogether, which is known as the *Valsalva technique*; this will create the most intense IAP. Too much IAP can also create a problem. The Valsalva technique can create so much IAP that weak cardiopulmonary systems might not tolerate the pressure. It has been documented that patients with weak hearts or high blood pressure must be careful when constipated because bearing down while holding their breath could result in a heart attack or a stroke.

When lifting weights, especially when powerlifting, you push out into your abdominal wall to create the greatest IAP.[10] Therefore, powerlifters often wear thick belts around their waist to aid in IAP while lifting. Less IAP is needed when dancing or swinging a golf club; hence, the need to push or pull is often an exaggeration. Some people get confused when we discuss core control, thinking that drawing in the abdominal wall is going to give them more stiffness or control. This is not true. The question that I pose is as follows: Is the competition to see who can generate the most IAP or who is the most efficient mover when the IAP is just enough?

As discussed in Chapter 4, the distribution of movement equals the distribution of force. Once we have adequate mobility for the functional task, we want to improve alignment and train control through the manipulation of load and tempo based on the activities in which the client chooses to participate; whether the client chooses to powerlift or to dance can result in very different program designs for conditioning.

Force couples can be defined by muscles or muscle groups exuding similar forces in opposite directions to increase stiffness and prepare for acceleration or deceleration of the extremities. The spine is no exception; the different layers of the trunk musculature that were explained previously can be considered a force couple. One of the examples I like to use is XX's. As discussed earlier, the anterior and posterior diagonal fascial slings create an X in front and an X in back. These elastic fascial slings are more effective when the abdominal and lumbar musculature work together to stiffen the elasticity that may be needed by the lower and upper extremities.

One of the more commonly discussed force couples is found in the shoulder girdle where the rotator cuff muscles approximate the head of the humerus into the glenoid fossa and improve the congruence of the joint, as discussed in Chapter 5. The force couple improving congruence now makes it possible for the primary movers (ie, the deltoid muscles) to do their job efficiently in movement of the upper extremity.

Another term used in learning movement is *neutral*. I prefer to use *optimal position* or *optimal placement* rather than neutral. This pertains to putting the joints in their optimal placement or alignment. How does one know where the optimal alignment is? Functionally, we can ask a client to move into the relative end of ranges within a plane of movement. Theoretically, in the middle of that range would be their optimal position today. That position will change over time as they improve their body awareness and tissues begin to adapt. One of the things that we often look at with this idea of optimal placement is understanding how different everyone is and how much variance there is in the normal human body.

Reality tells us that a neutral spine is a concept not a fixed position. For example, if a client has a large buttock and they are lying on their back for an exercise in which the anterior superior iliac spine and the pubic symphysis are used to establish a "neutral pelvis" in relation to the floor, this will put the lumbar spine in relative extension and, in some cases, hyperextension. If I asked them to lift their leg up at that time, that would put their back in a very precarious position and cause an anterior shear force. On the opposite side of the spectrum, when a client with no redundant tissue lies flat on their back, they might look like they are lying in neutral but have very limited range of motion in the sagittal plane. Everyone's body is different! Each person deserves a personalized assessment and program based on structure, strategy, and psychology.

For our purposes in this book, we are going to think of a neutral or optimal spine as being a concept in which the spine or spinal segments are in their middle range where there is the greatest potential for movement in all available planes as dictated by that motion segment. This does not imply that one must always maintain this posture. It is quite the opposite; it is the place where the greatest potential for movement or control of movement exists.

Another word that requires definition is stability. A lot of times we misinterpret stability. When I had my neck surgery, the surgeon came into my room right after surgery and said, "Brent, your neck is stable now." I was a bit taken aback as I laid there with a collar around my neck and titanium plates and 8 screws taking away all my ability to control the movement of my head. I was so out of it from the Dilaudid (hydromorphone) that I did not argue with the surgeon. I want to clarify that stability is the control of mobility. After my neck surgery, they fused 4 segments with a plate. There was no movement there; hence, there was no stability, only rigidity. Mobility must exist before any control can be exercised. This is true when we use examples in the financial or economic sense. We would say it is "economically stable," which means there is a balance between assets and debts. Likewise, in the ecosystem, what is a "stable ecosystem"? Again, it is a balance between prey and predators to maintain a stable natural habitat.

We know what an old pond looks like that has been stagnant for a long time; it is stinky, the fish are dead, and it is not a healthy place. Likewise, in our body, a stable pH is a balance between acidity and alkalinity, and a stable

body has to do with a balance of movement and stiffness. I like to use Manohar Panjabi's definition of stability, which is "the appropriate amount of stiffness for the anticipated load." Children learn this automatically and early in life with no external coaching or cueing to lift the pelvic floor or pull in their abdominals. Children do not do that, and neither should we. Our body learns how to anticipate load based on the activity we choose. Novel activity will often result in poor judgment, cocontractions, and over-recruitment because of unfamiliarity. Imagine a little child picking up a toy for the first time. They bend down to pick up their toy and fall on their face. The second time they go to pick up that toy, they think, "I did not like falling on my face; I would rather fall on my butt. I am going to put more weight posteriorly when I pick up that toy." Consequently, they fall on their diaper and realize that the diaper felt better than hitting their face on the ground, and then they start adjusting as they grow. By the time a child is 2 to 4 years old, they have it figured out. They spontaneously know what it is like to prepare themselves to pick things up and efficiently organize the neuromuscular system. This should be an automatic function that we have developed over the years. The problem is that when we get hurt or we sit for too long, we often disrupt the healthy patterns of organization where stability happens naturally and spontaneously. When we do not anticipate correctly, we end up having an imbalance of forces that leads to compensations, impaired movement, and, potentially, injury (Box 6-2).

Stability is the control of movement; it is the appropriate amount of stiffness for the anticipated load, with stiffness being used in a positive sense in which there is enough of a cocontraction around the involved joints to ensure that our movement is efficient and spontaneous. Let us return to the yoga concept of bandhas or cocontractions of joint complexes. As stated by Simon Borg-Olivier, bandhas protect the integrity of the noncontractile structures and force the load into the myofascial/contractile structures, which are much better at adapting to load.

BOX 6-2

At 10 years old, boys always have some trick up their sleeve. I was no different. My close childhood friends and I had the idea that it would be funny to use superglue to fix a quarter on the tiles in the mall and watch people try to pick it up. I am sure it was an idea that came from Candid Camera, one of my favorite childhood shows. We watched people break fingernails, trip, and even fall down. While we were laughing, the universe was taking notes. Some refer to this as karma.

Fast-forward 10 plus years to when I am with one of the same friends working for UPS at night emptying trucks while going to college. We had a weight restriction of 70 pounds (30 kg), which I was able to lift all night long. I had finished emptying a 40-ft (about 12-m) trailer, and I was feeling pretty proud of myself. I was just about to sweep out the trailer and close the door when I noticed a small box in the middle of the trailer. I ran back in and swooped down to pick it up. Little did I know that the box contained 70 or so pounds of lead pellets. I fell over and strained my back. Within a fraction of a second of the spectacle and my being completely surprised by the miscalculation of the weight of that small box, I had a flashback of the time that my friends and I glued a coin to the floor of the mall. Karma stunk that day.

Panjabi's model,[17,18] which is still the gold standard today, talks about stability consisting of 3 components: the neural control, the contractile tissues, and the noncontractile structures. The image used to depict the model uses a triangle with neural control at the tip and contractile (active) and noncontractile (inert) on the bottom corners. The noncontractile structures are the ligaments, the discs, the cartilage, and the bones (Figure 6-8). The contractile structures are the muscles and tendons, which are commonly referred to as *myofascial tissues* or *elastic tissues*, in response to the movement task. Panjabi stated that "when one of these functions is impaired, often it is accompanied by a dysfunction of the other two."[17,18] This can be observed in cases of low back pain. For instance, if someone injures a disc or ligament, they will have a motor control deficit that we call *pain inhibition*. This occurs when the local muscles that would normally provide the stiffness necessary to provide stability to the spine and prepare for multiplane movement are turned off as a protective mechanism. Then, they over-recruit the large global muscles that go into spasm and are often related to secondary pain from the original injury or pain mechanism. We can find the same phenomenon in shoulder injuries in which the rotator cuff is inhibited by pain, resulting in a lack of approximation of the joint and a similar over-recruitment of the global muscles around the joint. When the upper extremity is involved in overhead activity, the impingement is perturbed, and the cycle of impingement continues—pain, inhibition, impingement, and pain again. A good practitioner has to figure out how to inhibit the global muscle tone, wake up the local stabilizers, and evaluate if the integrity of the noncontractile structures is enough to avoid bracing or surgical intervention.

Pilates-based rehabilitation has been successful with rehabilitating low back pain.[4,19-25] I believe this is because of the unique tools in the Pilates environment that make it possible to manipulate alignment and load, resulting in a movement experience that positively shifts the movement-equals-pain paradigm. In the Pilates environment, a practitioner can introduce segmental movements (ie, small

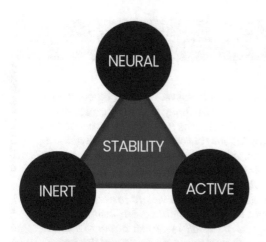

PANJABI'S MODEL OF STABILITY 1992

Figure 6-8. Panjabi's model of stability.

(Adapted from Panjabi MM. The stabilizing system of the spine. Part I. Function, dysfunction, adaptation, and enhancement. *J Spinal Disord*. 1992;5[4]:383-389; discussion 397.)

movements that are going to turn off the global stabilizers and wake up the local stabilizers). Within a couple sessions, the client can already determine if that awareness for those local stabilizers is enough for them to return to a healthy lifestyle. Many of these people avoid surgery and avoid interventions that would be very costly or potentially very risky to them. This is why I love using Pilates to treat people with low back pain.[4,19,22,24-27]

When we look at the noncontractile structures, we often look at the ligaments, capsules, and discs, also fully integrated with fascia, that control the joints of the spine. What we want to do is create this optimal orientation or alignment to restore mobility in the surrounding joints and tissues to minimize excessive forces and motion through injured or lax tissues. By changing the movement strategy and minimizing harmful forces, clients can often return to their normal activities of daily living, and in many cases, far exceed their expectations.

NEUTRAL ZONE

Another model of looking at spine organization, introduced by Panjabi[17,18] and later explained by Comerford and Mottram,[5,6] is the neutral zone. The neutral zone is a region of intervertebral motion around the neutral posture of a joint segment where little resistance is offered by the passive spinal column. As I mentioned previously, we want to keep that disc in a very healthy range and a healthy load. As a rule of thumb, we should always remember that injury occurs at end of range. Injury typically does not occur in midrange. The diagram in Figure 6-9 by Panjabi represents a schematic of end of range of motion.[18] The far left and far right of the graphic represent end of range of motion limited by noncontractile structures. This is where we have our greatest potential of injury. The space in the middle represents the neutral zone, which is where movement is controlled by subtle, subconscious contractions of the local stabilizers, maintaining enough stiffness to move safely through space. If an individual with a healthy body had options to move from 10 vertebral segments, they would likely never have to leave the neutral zone and still have a lot of movement range with great control, fluidity, and efficiency. However, if they only had 1 or 2 segments that they chose to move from in complex movements, they would leave the neutral zone and go toward the end of range of motion, which is where an injury of the disc and the ligaments is most likely to occur. This idea of the neutral zone can be applied to the extremities, as well as the axial skeleton. Let us return to an earlier concept in mobility—the distribution of movement equals the distribution of force. This will minimize the risk of injury to the noncontractile structure in their end of range. For a client with a knee pathology, a simple solution is to redirect the focus of intervention to increase the mobility of the hip and ankle in weight-bearing strategies. Apply the bone rhythm strategies to the lower extremity to create new successful movement experiences without pain.

The neuromuscular factors are the essential components of maintaining the neutral zone within normal limits. The multifidus and other deep local stabilizers are essential to provide control of the motion segment, providing greater than two-thirds of the stiffness increase in the L4-5 and L5-S1 segments and preventing shear forces and abnormal movements that again would lead over time to trauma to the discs, ligaments, facets, and degenerative changes.[28]

CORE CONTROL

Core control is often misunderstood in today's vernacular. Many think it is the same thing as having a strong abdominal wall. Control is not equivalent to strength. Control is when you have the appropriate tension or compression for the desired movement. If I were a Cirque du Soleil performer, I might have my spine moving in all different positions and have a tremendous amount of stiffness at certain points of time in certain segments to be able to safely perform the movement. This inner unit, according to Diane Lee,[29,30] must be able to create the appropriate amount of stiffness at a segmental level. Endurance and strength are achieved with practice and are not to be minimized.

If I recruit too many muscles or think that I must recruit this powerhouse every time that I move, I am going to get in my own way. I learned from one of my great mentors, Dr. Alan Lee, "as much as necessary as little as possible." I have a feeling that Dr. Lee got this saying from Confucius. This goes back to what Pilates and the Feldenkrais Method teach pertaining to the efficiency of movement.[1] Joseph Pilates stated that we should perform our many varied daily tasks naturally and spontaneously.[1] We should not be thinking: *Is my powerhouse drawn in while I am bending down to pick up my child?* No, it is something natural that we anticipate correctly because we understand the tasks from the history of our many subconscious, goal-driven, and positive movement experiences. The other thing I want to mention is that the muscular slings

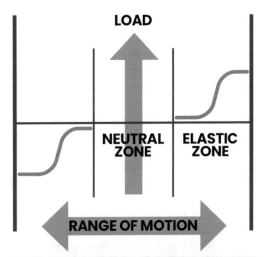

SPINAL STABILITY CONCEPT

Figure 6-9. The neutral zone according to Panjabi.

(Reproduced with permission from Panjabi MM. The stabilizing system of the spine. Part II. Neutral zone and instability hypothesis. *J Spinal Disord.* 1992;5[4]:390-396.)

will engage appropriately, and their activation is dictated by the movement and load itself, not by us telling them to contract.[2,13,31] When our body moves, the myofascial tissue feels the strain and communicates to the body what muscles need to prepare in anticipation of that movement. More recently, the fascial system has been considered the largest proprioceptive organ in the body.[2] It is filled with Golgi organs, which are thought to be our mechanoreceptors that are sensitive to gravity and uprightness. This becomes very exciting. When we have proper postural organization (ie, axial elongation), we rely more on the tensile organization of the connective tissue, like a child, and the proprioceptive system will automatically respond to the load, creating the appropriate amount of tension/elasticity/control/stability. The attention should be focused on alignment, axial length, mobility, load, and creating successful movement experiences, not on a muscle contraction of the core. As we vary the load, we can facilitate the natural neuromuscular organization.

PROPRIOCEPTION

As I mentioned previously in this chapter, the multifidi, in their normal organization, play a very important role in proprioception of the spine. According to Bogduk and Twomey,[28] the multifidus contains 6 times the number of muscle spindle fibers compared with the rest of the muscles of the spine. The muscle spindle fiber is a contractile fiber embedded in the muscle and provides a sensory component that communicates with the central nervous system in the spine. It can communicate how much load is coming through that muscle, as well as the segmental posture and its orientation with gravity and load. The efficiency of the local stabilizers around the spine can be trained to be more efficient through movement awareness training. The focus on "as much as necessary as little as possible" can continue to improve motor efficiencies vs volitionally creating something that interferes with normal healthy movement planning. Another proprioceptor being discussed more recently is the Golgi organ found in the fascia. Current research shows an abundance of Golgi organ receptors in the fascia where its primary focus is related to axial alignment of the body against gravity. These receptors are trainable to create unconscious competence in our posture and movement strategies, returning the pleasure and zest to movement.

INTRA-ABDOMINAL PRESSURE

The TA, and its normal organization, is thought to increase IAP as appropriate for the anticipated load. In healthy participants, Hodges and Richardson[8,32] looked at how the TA and the other abdominal muscles responded in anticipation of movement of the arm. In a flexion, abduction, and extension moment, they identified a very interesting phenomenon in which the TA fired 50 milliseconds before the firing of the deltoid of the arm when instructed to lift the arm over the head or out to the side. The TA consistently performed 50 milliseconds before the firing of the primary mover in the healthy participants. A 50-millisecond anticipatory response is a subconscious and subcortical contraction. In a low back pain population in the same study, Hodges showed that the participants with low back pain did not have a consistent firing of the TA 50 milliseconds before the firing of the primary mover. Even the fastest volitional contractions of muscles are thought to be somewhere between 250 and 500 milliseconds. The TA fires at 50 milliseconds before the contraction of the primary muscle firing to move the limb, which is 5 to 6 times faster than a volitional contraction.

Many extrapolated the research of Hodges and Richardson, listed before, and insinuated that performing volitional training of the TA will return the TA to its normal function in individuals with low back pain. This does not seem to have any advantage over any other exercise or movement training for patients with low back pain. Even in severe cases in which the rehabilitation warrants isolation training of the abdominal muscles, the exercises need to be progressed to the level where the neuromuscular system responds spontaneously to load. I find quite often, through alignment and load training, that volitional training of TA contraction is not necessary to restore function (Box 6-3).

The other thing Hodges[8,32] discovered was that it was a subthreshold contraction, meaning that it was probably in the 30% range of its maximum voluntary contraction. We are going to have a sense of being prepared for a movement, but we are not going to feel a strong maximal voluntary contraction of the muscles as in the previous experiment of volitionally contracting the core muscles compared with an image of axial length. How free did you feel when you had the image of axial length using the balloons between the vertebra and you recruited just enough tone appropriate for the desired movement? Our body works with subthreshold or submaximal contraction all the time. The pelvic floor muscles also respond

BOX 6-3: SPONTANEOUS VERSUS VOLITIONAL ACTIVATION EXPERIMENT

Volitional: Standing on both feet shoulder-width apart, draw the abdominal muscles in and lift the pelvic floor muscles at the same time. Once the core muscles are activated, rotate the axial skeleton around the central axis. Observe how it feels. Is it an efficient use of energy?

Spontaneous: Now, in the same stance, imagine that between each spinal vertebra the disc is like a balloon or inner tube. Let all the air out of the discs so that the spine collapses into flexion. Imagine that there is a pump that now fills each of the balloons or inner tubes with air, stacking the spine into its optimal position. Now, rotate the axial skeleton around the central axis. Observe how it feels. Now, imagine that you have a gallon or 2 liters of water in each hand. How does the body react? Maybe even increase the imagined weight to 10 kilos or 24 pounds in each hand; what happens now? Finally, imagine releasing the weights in the hand and continuing to spiral around the central axis.

Compare the 2 strategies of trunk control. Hopefully, you observed that the spontaneous approach was more efficient than the volitional and that the volitional contractions interfered with the ease of the movement. Even when we imagined carrying load in our arms, the reaction was a slight increase in tone and possibly a decrease in the range of motion.

to IAP with subconscious, subthreshold contractions to maintain the integrity of the IAP needed for the desired task. The pelvic floor muscles and diaphragm work harmoniously with the core wall muscles.

The hydraulic amplifier model helps us understand that when the diaphragm contracts and descends, it will increase the IAP (see Figure 3-5 in Chapter 3). If the task at hand only requires a specific amount of IAP, then the TA and the pelvic floor muscles are going to eccentrically contract to aid in the regulation of the IAP. Upon exhalation, the diaphragm relaxes and elastically ascends, reducing the IAP unless the demand from the task requires the TA and the pelvic floor muscles to concentrically contract to sustain the IAP while the diaphragm relaxes.

STIFFNESS VERSUS MOBILITY

The last part of this idea of faulty organization and the motor control aspect of the spine as it pertains to axial length is achieving a balance between stiffness and mobility. This is something that we learn over time, and everyone is different. If we drew a bell curve and assessed the range of stiffness from healthy mobile to healthy stiff, more than 90% of the population would fall within the normal bell curve (Figure 6-10). Some people would say "I'm so stiff," whereas others would say "I am so hypermobile." Our objective in treatment is to approximate toward the center of the curve to achieve our ideal balance between stiffness and mobility. Stability is the appropriate amount of control over the mobility necessary to execute a desired task.

STANDARD DEVIATIONS

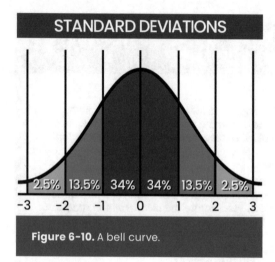

| 2.5% | 13.5% | 34% | 34% | 13.5% | 2.5% |

-3   -2   -1   0   1   2   3

Figure 6-10. A bell curve.

Stolze et al[19] published their research in the *Journal of Orthopaedic & Sports Physical Therapy*. Lise Stolze, a physical therapist, Pilates teacher, and a Polestar educator, was looking at the predictive rule of how Pilates can affect people with mechanical low back pain. These prediction rules can identify subgroups of patients with low back pain who are most likely to benefit from Pilates-based exercise. It helps us understand which patients will respond best to movement education vs manual therapies or surgery. What other factors pertaining to the individual will best predict the individual's outcome? Stolze et al found several factors that help predict which patients will get better with Pilates intervention alone. Some of these factors include being overweight, having a high body fat percentage of total body weight, and having localized low back pain without symptoms below the knee. The predictability rule proposed by Stolze et al and other studies are beginning to help us explain why so many people with low back pain improve with movement therapies such as Pilates.[4,19,33] When we place a spine in its optimal position and give it the appropriate amount of stiffness, it has the greatest chance of healing and performing well while at the same time minimizing the forces that perturb the original lesion. It does not mean that some people are not going to need surgery because they will. What it means is that we minimize the risk. We optimize performance.

FEAR OF PAIN

Fear is also a significant factor in compensation and can interfere with normal movement strategies. When we incur an injury to a noncontractile structure, such as the disc, capsule, ligament, muscle, or bone, we experience a neurologic inhibition, which is usually due to pain and perceived danger or the risk of incurring more tissue damage. Pain will often result in a local inhibition of the local/deep stabilizer muscles. The deep muscles (eg, the rotator cuff, deep hip rotators, multifidi, medial fibers of the psoas and quadratus lumborum, and TA) will often be inhibited. This increases the exposure and range of the neutral zone, increasing the vulnerability to excessive forces. This often results in a functional instability and vulnerability to the smallest of movements that can create pain. Simple things like a sneeze, bending down to tie your shoes, or putting your pants on can stimulate pain excitation. The body will compensate for the pain by splinting, and the fear will prevent the individual from moving because of the anticipation of pain occurring. To prevent that, the body, or the mind, sends a signal to recruit the global stabilizers. The global stabilizers consist of the deltoids, the quadratus lumborum, the erector spinae, the psoas major, and the piriformis, to name a few. These muscles go into a spasm or overcompensate, but because they are not endurance muscles, they fatigue very quickly and become very painful. People associate movement with pain, and the result is fear to move. One thing we can do is to create positive movement experiences that teach them that movement equals happiness. By having these positive movement experiences without pain, they can start believing and having hope again that they can be restored to normal movement and not have to deal with pain for the rest of their life. If they have enough of these positive movement experiences, they can overcome their pain. We can do this by waking up the local stabilizers and inhibiting the global stabilizers. By applying the principles of mobility, breath, and axial elongation, we can facilitate segmental movement in a controlled environment, a safe environment, and a safe range of motion, awakening the local stabilizers and inhibiting the global stabilizers. Simple movements, including bridging, a pelvic clock, or a spring-assisted extremity movement, can start to wake up the local stabilizers almost immediately and increase the feeling of well-being. We see people within 2 or 3 sessions after a mechanical back injury already feeling 60% to 80% better with a marked decrease in the fear of movement.

FAULTY MOVEMENT PATTERNS

Some people ask the following question: "What are some of the reasons for faulty movement organization?" I have categorized the answer into 3 areas: genetic predisposition, habitual patterns, and compensatory patterns. The first is genetic predisposition (ie, familial traits of the musculoskeletal system and how our bodies are organized). Some people might have a leg-length discrepancy, scoliosis, or other genetic predispositions, such as a family history of spine disease. Physical anomalies do exist, and in these cases, we follow Eric Franklin's definition of ideal posture—"optimal alignment is when the body structures come in as close to the central axis as structure permits and the center of gravity as low as structure permits."[34] The beauty of this definition is that everyone can still have optimal alignment. We do the best we can with a body that has significant redundancy, neuroplasticity, and hope.

The second area is habitual patterns; I think this is probably the most common cause of faulty movement patterns. Sitting is probably one of the worst habitual patterns that affects our body's ability to participate in healthy normal movement. We often sit with our legs crossed or assume a slouched posture. Gaming has become a major pastime for our youth and young adults. Our youth are spending on average 13 hours per day sitting

in slouched positions. We can also add to the list our habits of driving, sleeping, and carrying boxes or backpacks. Even in sports, we can identify asymmetrical organization that defines your sporting activity and even the position you play on a soccer team or the race you run in track. With a lot of experience working with dancers, I always find it entertaining to guess what style of dance they practice or who they studied under before they tell me. If they practice ballet, modern dance, ethnic dance, tap, or jazz or were on Broadway, their bodies have adapted to the activities they practice. Another Eric Franklin saying is "We are what we practice." Our body will look like what we practice. Our habits depict what we look like. Most body awareness exercises are neutral in their ability to optimize our ability to move naturally and spontaneously through our many daily activities. These movement forms can also neutralize some of the negative effects found in asymmetrical activities. If we have a client with a bias of external rotation in their hips as a ballet dancer, we will emphasize working in hip neutral and internal rotation to balance the asymmetry. Even the clothes we wear can create habitual changes to our posture and motor plans (eg, high-heeled shoes, baggy pants sagging around the upper thighs, hip huggers, tight pencil skirts). Fashion can play havoc on our bodies if we let it. Habitual patterns are in all of us. We all need to find movement forms and exercises that have a balancing and neutralizing effect on our daily habits to optimize performance. It is as simple as that. The question is how do we modify a behavior that we are doing 13 hours a day with a few exercises?

The third area is compensatory patterns. As a physical therapist, I see them all the time. I will have a patient come in and say "My shoulder is really hurting, can you take a look at it?" So, I look at the shoulder, I fix the shoulder, and they come back the next day and say "My shoulder feels a lot better, but funny enough I have a pain here in my neck that I had 6 months ago." After the neck is fixed, they come back and say "Oh, my shoulder and neck are feeling better, but my right sacroiliac is hurting now. That is a problem I had about 2 years ago." It is like an onion; we have to peel away the layers. These are all compensatory patterns. Every time we have an injury, we tend to develop a compensatory pattern to be able to heal and protect ourselves. However, not all compensatory patterns are bad; many of them are necessary for us to function. We use this all the time in neurologic rehabilitation.

Function needs to be the primary goal. The client's awareness of compensatory strategies provides a great place to begin education for the client's behavior shift. It is possible to facilitate good alignment, organization, control, and efficiency that will help eliminate some of these harmful compensatory strategies that tend to get in the way of healing. The following is an example of this. If I have hip pain and I compensate by minimizing hip extension through a hip flexor strategy, every time I toe-off while walking, the shortened hip flexors will create a shear force on the lumbar spine. I might not notice that my hip flexor is tight, but then I start having back pain and maybe even stenotic symptoms from repetitive strain related to the shear force in my lower back. Before we can help the lower back pain, we need to restore hip extension.

To reiterate, compensatory patterns can be normal and healthy, but they can also be problematic and lead to other problems. Compensatory patterns can also be caused by psychological or emotional challenges, with fear of movement being the greatest psychosocial factor. No matter the movement form (ie, tai chi, yoga, Gyrotonic Expansion System, Pilates, qigong, Feldenkrais Method, or other martial arts and dance forms), they all have a goal of bringing awareness between the body, mind, and spirit.

BIOENERGETICS

We want to understand the flow, balance, and control of energy, especially as they relate to human movement. When we reference chi or prana flowing through our bodies, we are often referring to a source or centering of life's energy (eg, the root chakra located in the pelvic region or the crown chakra located on the top of the head). This energy can be directed through the body with breathing techniques, mantras, and of course, movement. Many times in whole body movement, we are literally moving the whole body (ie, all the systems). I remember very early on when I was learning Pilates, I would take time in the evening to practice Pilates through a different system of the body. I would distinguish the influence movement had over the various systems of the body, including the skeletal, muscular, nervous, pulmonary, digestive, and circulatory systems. Years later, I went back and experienced Pilates through a more energetic assessment. I would ask myself what happens to chi as I moved my body in a rollover or a roll up or into an extension? How does my breath change? As I observed movement in clients and students, I noticed that when they would hold their breath or lose axial elongation in their movements (eg, the swan), it would result in a very different manifestation of energy in their faces and throughout their body compared with someone who was very fluid and had mastered relaxation, breath, and fluidity with their movement. The latter had a glow of energy around their head, neck, and shoulders and space.

As our understanding of the fascial system deepens, we are realizing that the fascia is a major energy source and communication tool for the body; some even refer to it as *collective consciousness*. Recent research of the fascial Golgi organs shows they are responsible for upright postural alignment. In Western medicine, we still struggle to understand that a good flow of energy can be related to what Chinese medicine teaches through the meridians and the flow of chi. One of the foundations in Chinese medicine is the flow of chi; if the chi is balanced, then the body will heal itself. It is different from Western medicine where we just want the pill or surgery that is going to cure us.

When we move well, I believe we create an effect similar to something like acupuncture, freeing up the flow of chi and energy through our body. Our body is in a better state to heal itself and to be healthier overall. The principle of control, stimulated by varying loads, is a powerful tool that facilitates health, awareness, and stability in our lives.

OPEN-ENDED QUESTIONS

1 Explain how the local stabilizing muscles of the trunk provide the appropriate amount of stiffness for the anticipated load. Where is the neurocontrol center for the local stabilizers?

2 How does the myofascial tissue provide trunk support and stability during movement? Explain the fascial lines that directly relate to human movements.

3 Discuss how the multifidi, psoas major, quadratus lumborum, transverse abdominus, oblique muscles, pelvic floor, and diaphragm all interact subconsciously with the connective fascia to maintain dynamic control.

4 Explain how dynamic alignment influences the spontaneous muscle contractions necessary to facilitate stability. How can axial alignment facilitate greater movement efficiency in most upright activities?

5 How can a design of an exercise with good alignment demand spontaneous organization?

6 Define in your own words what a closed kinetic chain is and how it works. Give examples of exercises that incorporate closed chain activities.

7 Define in your own words what an open kinetic chain is and how it works. Give examples of exercises that incorporate closed chain activities.

8 Define in your own words what a pseudo-closed kinetic chain is and how it works. Give examples of exercises that incorporate closed chain activities.

9 How can you differentiate between the right amount of IAP and too much or too little IAP?

10 How does one know when they are teaching the right amount of IAP to match the load?

OPEN-ENDED QUESTIONS

11 Describe how the force couple of the rotator cuff works to optimize upper extremity movement. How does the rotator cuff work during functional overhead tasks and at the same time avoid subacromial impingement?

12 Explain why different individuals can have what appears to be variations to the traditional definition of a neutral pelvis in relation to the spine in supine and yet both be in a functional or optimal neutral posture.

13 Share a modern definition of stability; look for similarities regarding a stable economy, ecosystem, structures, and emotional well-being. Incorporate the concept of balance into your definition.

14 Describe how anticipatory load works; how do we as humans learn to anticipate load? How do children learn to anticipate load? Give examples of a toddler learning movement tasks.

15 Explain how you would help a client in a compensatory pattern of local inhibition and global excitation wake up the deep local stabilizing muscles and inhibit the muscles in spasm. Hint: Think of the principle of mobility.

16 Describe how graded load can be used to progress a client that is unable to tolerate the full load of their normal daily activities and tasks. How do you determine what is the appropriate load?

17 Define the "neutral zone" in your own words. Expand on the difference of the neutral zone compared to core control, which have often been discussed in the literature over the past 30 years.

18 Describe how providing a successful movement experience without pain can help reverse the effects of secondary guarding and inhibition as seen in fear-of-pain protection. Where is the control center to wake up the local stabilizers that have been shut off?

19 Describe how the deep local muscles in the low back contain a high ratio of muscle spindle fibers. How can the reawakening of the deep local muscles affect the proprioception of the axial skeleton?

20 List an example of each type of faulty movement pattern: genetic, habitual, and compensatory. Hypothesize how your treatment or training approach to restore function might differ for each.

REFERENCES

1. Pilates JH, Robbins J, Van Heuit-Robbins L. *Pilates Evolution: The 21st Century*. Presentation Dynamics; 2012.

2. Schleip R, Baker A, Avison J. *Fascia in Sport and Movement*. Handspring Publishing; 2015.

3. Ingber DE. The architecture of life. *Sci Am*. 1998;278(1):48-57.

4. Anderson BD. *Randomized Clinical Trial Comparing Active Versus Passive Approaches to the Treatment of Recurrent and Chronic Low Back Pain* [dissertation]. University of Miami; 2005.

5. Comerford MJ, Mottram SL. Movement and stability dysfunction—contemporary developments. *Man Ther*. 2001;6(1):15-26.

6. Comerford MJ, Mottram SL. Functional stability re-training: principles and strategies for managing mechanical dysfunction. *Man Ther*. 2001;6(1):3-14.

7. Hodges P, Heijnen I, Gandevia SC. Postural activity of the diaphragm is reduced in humans when respiratory demand increases. *J Physiol*. 2001;537(Pt 3):999-1008.

8. Hodges PW, Richardson CA. Inefficient muscular stabilization of the lumbar spine associated with low back pain. A motor control evaluation of transversus abdominis. *Spine (Phila Pa 1976)*. 1996;21(22):2640-2650.

9. Lederman E. The fall of the postural-structural-biomechanical model in manual and physical therapies: exemplified by lower back pain. *J Bodyw Mov Ther*. 2011;15(2):131-138.

10. McGill S. *Low Back Disorders: Evidence-Based Prevention and Rehabilitation*. 2nd ed. Human Kinetics; 2007.

11. Norris C. Spinal stabilisation—1. active lumbar stabilisation—2. Limiting factors to end-range of motion in the lumbar spine—3. Stabilisation mechanisms of the lumbar spine. *Physiother J*. 1995;81(2):61-79.

12. Earls J. *Born to Walk: Myofascial Efficiency and the Body in Movement*. North Atlantic Books; 2014.

13. Myers TW. *Anatomy Trains: Myofascial Meridians for Manual and Movement Therapists*. 3rd ed. Elsevier; 2014.

14. Schleip R. *Fascia: The Tensional Network of the Human Body: The Science and Clinical Applications in Manual and Movement Therapy*. Churchill Livingstone/Elsevier; 2012.

15. Borg-Olivier S. *Applied Anatomy & Physiology of Yoga*. Warisanoffset.com; 2006.

16. Hewitt J. *The Complete Yoga Book: Yoga of Breathing, Yoga of Posture, and Yoga of Meditation*. Schocken Books; 1978.

17. Panjabi MM. The stabilizing system of the spine. Part II. Neutral zone and instability hypothesis. *J Spinal Disord*. 1992;5(4):390-396; discussion 397.

18. Panjabi MM. The stabilizing system of the spine. Part I. Function, dysfunction, adaptation, and enhancement. *J Spinal Disord*. 1992;5(4):383-389; discussion 397.

19. Stolze LR, Allison SC, Childs JD. Derivation of a preliminary clinical prediction rule for identifying a subgroup of patients with low back pain likely to benefit from Pilates-based exercise. *J Orthop Sports Phys Ther*. 2012;42(5):425-436.

20. Cruz-Ferreira A, Fernandes J, Laranjo L, Bernardo LM, Silva A. A systematic review of the effects of pilates method of exercise in healthy people. *Arch Phys Med Rehabil*. 2011;92(12):2071-2081.

21. Black M, Calais-Germain B, Vleeming A. *Centered: Organizing the Body Through Kinesiology, Movement Theory and Pilates Technique*. Handspring Publishing; 2015.

22. Caldwell K, Adams M, Quin R, Harrison M, Greeson J. Pilates, mindfulness and somatic education. *J Dance Somat Pract*. 2013;5(2):141-153.

23. Garcia-Soidan JL, Giraldez VA, Cachon Zagalaz J, Lara-Sanchez AJ. Does pilates exercise increase physical activity, quality of life, latency, and sleep quantity in middle-aged people? *Percept Mot Skills*. 2014;119(3):838-850.

24. Vieira FT, Faria LM, Wittmann JI, Teixeira W, Nogueira LA. The influence of Pilates method in quality of life of practitioners. *J Bodyw Mov Ther*. 2013;17(4):483-487.

25. Yu KK, Tulloch E, Hendrick P. Interrater reliability of a Pilates movement-based classification system. *J Bodyw Mov Ther*. 2015;19(1):160-176.

26. Coleman TJ, Nygaard IE, Holder DN, Egger MJ, Hitchcock R. Intra-abdominal pressure during Pilates: unlikely to cause pelvic floor harm. *Int Urogynecol J*. 2015;26(8):1123-1130.

27. Priebe S, Savill M, Reininghaus U, et al. Effectiveness and cost-effectiveness of body psychotherapy in the treatment of negative symptoms of schizophrenia—a multi-centre randomised controlled trial. *BMC Psychiatry*. 2013;13:26.

28. Bogduk N, Twomey LT. *Clinical Anatomy of the Lumbar Spine*. Churchill Livingstone; 1987.

29. Lee D, Delta Orthopaedic Physiotherapy Clinic. *Manual Therapy for the Thorax: A Biomechanical Approach*. DOPC; 1994.

30. Lee D, Hodges PW. Behavior of the linea alba during a curl-up task in diastasis rectus abdominis: an observational study. *J Orthop Sports Phys Ther*. 2016;46(7):580-589.

31. Earls J, Myers TW. *Fascial Release for Structural Balance*. North Atlantic Books; 2010.

32. Richardson C, Hodges PW, Hides J. *Therapeutic Exercise for Lumbopelvic Stabilisation: A Motor Control Approach for the Treatment and Prevention of Low Back Pain*. 2nd ed. Churchill Livingstone; 2004.

33. Pereira LM, Obara K, Dias JM, et al. Comparing the Pilates method with no exercise or lumbar stabilization for pain and functionality in patients with chronic low back pain: systematic review and meta-analysis. *Clin Rehabil*. 2012;26(1):10-20.

34. Franklin EN. *Conditioning for Dance*. Human Kinetics; 2004.

MOVEMENT INTEGRATION

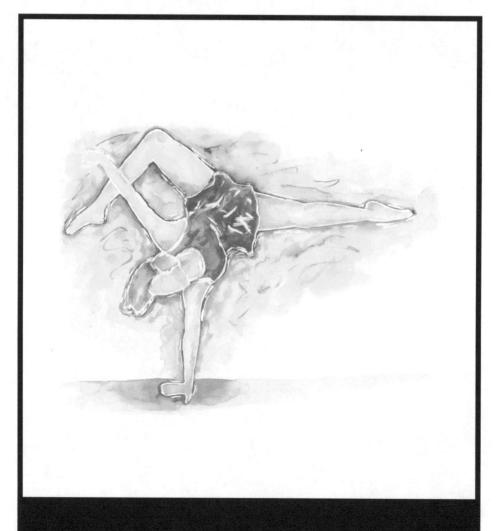

CREATE THE POSITIVE MOVEMENT EXPERIENCE WITHOUT PAIN, THAT EXCEEDS THEIR EXPECTATION.

CHAPTER OBJECTIVES

1 Learn to create positive movement experiences through the application and integration of the Principles of Movement.

2 Understand neuroplasticity and neuromuscular adaptation, and how the body adapts to images, thoughts, beliefs, load, and practice.

3 Create a movement learning strategy that likely will result in natural and spontaneous movement.

4 Understand and apply the science of motor control at a large scale, addressing movement from the individual's needs and beliefs, the desired task, and the environmental constraints that influence the individual's capacity.

5 Understand, at a basic level, different motor control theories and how they can be applied to movement acquisition. Apply the different theories based on the needs of the client.

6 Integrate the many different motor learning theories into movement instruction.

7 Acknowledge the impact successful movement can have on the psychosocial aspects of one's life. Learn how awareness and qualitative movement can greatly enhance the quality of life.

KEY TERMS

- Action
- Activities
- Associative learning
- Awareness
- Belief
- Classical conditioning
- Cognition
- Declarative learning
- Discrete vs continuous tasks
- Environment factors
- Extrinsic feedback
- Habituation
- Impairments
- International Classification of Functioning, Disability and Health
- Intrinsic feedback
- Mindfulness
- Motor learning
- Motor theory
- Movement integration
- Nonassociative learning
- Open vs closed tasks
- Operant conditioning
- Participation
- Perception
- Procedural learning
- Secondary gains
- Self-actualize
- Sensitization
- Stable vs mobile surfaces
- Strategic
- Tasks

Anderson BD.
Principles of Movement (pp 150-171).
© 2024 Taylor & Francis Group.

Movement integration is the principle that synthesizes all the Principles of Movement. It gives us the tools and understanding of new movement acquisition and learning new strategies to replace older and less efficient strategies. As we better understand the science of motor control and motor learning, we start to use a different set of tools than what might traditionally be used in the fitness, athletic, and rehabilitation sciences. We can define the task clearly in the environment that our clients choose to participate in, and we can successfully plan and facilitate their movement journey. Putting into practice the movement integration principle allows us to take into consideration certain limitations, faulty movement patterns, and the history of the client. How do we create positive movement experiences through the manipulation of the environment to shift the belief and hope patterns of the client so they can perform at their most effective level? As much as I appreciate the power in each of the movement principles, movement integration excites me the most. It allows us to understand neuroplasticity and how what we see is not always what is really underlying the movement challenges. It allows our minds to think beyond flexibility and strength training and rely on the other principles to facilitate proper mobility, control, coordination, efficiency, and perception. These all lead to very powerful outcome measures related to the client's perception of their abilities. This last principle helps us to better understand the vastness pertaining to movement in those who are healthy and those who are challenged with physical, neurologic, and psychosocial limitations.

CREATE THE POSITIVE MOVEMENT EXPERIENCE WITHOUT PAIN, THAT EXCEEDS THEIR EXPECTATION.

Movement integration is the final principle that synthesizes all the Principles of Movement. It is the pièce de résistance! It brings the acquisition of skill, efficiency, and awareness to daily tasks and functional activities. For movement integration to be optimized, we must have efficient breathing, mobility, good awareness and control, axial elongation, alignment, and load tolerance.

In addition, the impact of the mind and spirit, which for the purposes of this book, I refer to as belief, mindfulness, and awareness of self and surroundings, should be considered if we are to truly understand and apply the Principles of Movement holistically. Dawn Strom said, "The movement of the mind is reflected in the movement of the body, and the movement of the body in the mind. To move is to develop strength of this dynamic relationship between the mind, body, and the living synergy of one's environment."[1] In addition, Bonnie Bainbridge Cohen stated, "Our body moves as our mind moves. The qualities of movement are a manifestation of how the mind is expressing through the body at any moment ... movement can be a way to observe the expression of the mind through the body, and it can also be a way to affect change in the body-mind relationship."[2] There is a phrase in Proverbs that says, "For as he thinketh in his heart, so is he" (Proverbs 23:7). René Descartes brought a slightly different view with his statement, "I think, therefore I am." More modern interpretations found in the book *The Untethered Soul: The Journey Beyond Yourself* by Michael A. Singer challenge the idea of defining self by our thoughts; rather, Singer encourages defining self as the observer and in control of what thoughts we keep and what thoughts we eliminate or allow to pass away.[3] This ties in nicely with the recent science of neuroplasticity. We can say that our perception is our reality. One of the things we notice in the practice of mindful movement is the effect it can have on a person's perception of their well-being. Abraham Maslow's hierarchy of needs is a 5-tiered psychological model based on human needs and motivation. The levels represent physiological needs, safety, love and belonging, esteem, and self-actualization, respectfully. The 4 bottom levels are what he referred to as *deficiency needs*. The top tier is what he referred to as a *growth need*. Maslow's hierarchy of needs teaches us that if our most basic needs are not satisfied (eg, air, water, food, sleep), then it is difficult to attend to needs higher up.[4] Movement plays an important role in many of the basic needs, such as health, survival, and safety. Movement can also influence higher needs, including self-esteem and self-awareness, found in the fourth level. This is often a result of experiencing successful movements without pain or that exceed our expectations. If we can create successful movement experiences and build the perception of confidence in our client's movement, it can significantly impact one's well-being. Joseph Pilates took postural alignment, self-esteem, and confidence very seriously.[5,6] He believed that if movement could shift one's sense of health, strength, confidence, and self-esteem, it would directly impact a much bigger quest that we all have—to be happy. When we increase our awareness of our posture, exercise mental discipline, and establish a behavior of practice, we become more conscious of a uniformly developed mind, body, and spirit and are prepared to explore our higher selves and maximize our potential, or as Maslow said, "self-actualize."[4]

Successful movement integration requires that the individual gains a level of consciousness of their body, be it positive or negative in the beginning. Becoming aware of how our bodies move while performing a range of simple to complex tasks prepares the mind and body to consciously make a change. You cannot choose to change if you lack awareness of what needs to be changed. Movement never occurs in only one plane or a single body part. Even the simplest human movements (eg, walking, opening a door, picking up our children) are multiplanar, multidirectional complex movements. We take most of our daily movements for granted. When was the last time you thought about how to comb your hair or climb a set of stairs? For many of us, we go through our day performing these movements at a subconscious, natural, and spontaneous level unless we suffer an impairment that requires us to relearn the task. Joseph Pilates said, "Our interpretation of physical fitness is the attainment and maintenance of a uniformly developed body with a sound mind fully capable of naturally, easily, and satisfactorily performing our many and varied daily tasks with spontaneous zest and pleasure."[5]

MOTOR CONTROL

Motor control is the ability to regulate or direct the mechanisms essential to movement.[7] It deals with how the central nervous system organizes the many muscles and joints into functional movement. According to Anne Shumway-Cook and and Marjorie Woollacott, movement emerges from the interaction of 3 factors: the individual, the task, and the environment. Movement is both task-specific and constrained by the environment. The individual moves to meet the demands of the tasks within the constraints of the environment. The ability to move according to the task and environment constraints determines the individual's functional capacity[7] (Figure 7-1). The first aspect of motor control to address for the purposes of this chapter is the individual. Within the individual, movement arises from the interaction of multiple processes, including those that are related to perception, cognition, and action.[7] The World Health Organization's model for the classification of

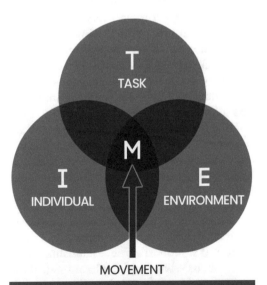

Figure 7-1. The motor control theory model.

(Reproduced with permission from Shumway-Cook AW, Woollacott MH. *Motor Control Theory and Practical Applications*. 2nd ed. Lippincott Williams & Wilkins; 2001.)

movement impairments defines the severity by the individual's inability to perform normal daily tasks as basic as standing, sitting, walking, jumping, reaching, speaking, rolling, and even smiling. In the science of motor control, we ask the following questions: (1) Where and how is that task controlled? and (2) Is it a pattern located in the spinal cord, or is it generated as a novel movement in the brain through a desire to perform a task (eg, a baby feeding itself for the first time)? It takes into consideration the many factors that influence human movement, which are often referred to as the *degrees of freedom*. Movement is defined as human actions or tasks, whereas motor control is defined as the science that tries to identify how the many degrees of freedom are controlled pertaining to human actions.[8] Let us explore the processes of perception, cognition, and action.

Perception is one of my favorite topics. It played a very large part in my research, specifically how people perceived their ability to perform.[9-11] Perception is the integration of sensory impressions into psychologically meaningful information.[7] If the sensory system sends signals to the brain and the brain perceives pain, then it can influence movement control or the lack thereof. This can also be explained with body awareness pertaining to posture and its relationship to the environment around it. The senses of vision, proprioception, and even smell can affect action. For example, when you smell freshly baked chocolate chip cookies, you may think that they smell good, and immediately your perception influences your actions.

Cognition broadly includes attention, motivation, and emotional aspects of motor control that underlie the establishment of intent or goals. Now that you have smelled the cookie, you have acknowledged the perception that this is something good. Then, your brain says "This is something that I want." It is going to have you take action. As you walk over to the kitchen, you realize that you must kiss your mother and say hello to her before you can indulge in the cookie. Because the motivation is still present, cognitively you are solving the problems before you to get to the desired cookie or to take action (ie, the third aspect of the individual).

Action is what the body does in response to the cognitive strategy to get that cookie (ie, walking over, bending over, kissing your mother, reaching for the cookie, and putting the cookie in your mouth). Action for most adults is spontaneous, and the body responds to the desired task. I know this can be a little overwhelming, but it is essential to truly understand movement. Another way of understanding this aspect of the individual can be framed as follows: The senses provide awareness (perception) of what is happening around us. These senses create a thought or a goal of a task (cognitive). This goal is executed (action) through the body to achieve the desired goal.

In another scenario, if a client is afraid of falling and they perceive something as a risk, whether it really is a risk or not, that belief then contributes to the cognitive process influencing their ability to move. Their body might react negatively by over-recruiting muscles, leading to an increased risk of falling. Falling becomes a negative motivation and eventually can lead to a loss of desire to move or participate at all. Contrary to this scenario, when we provide individuals who have a high risk of falling with a positive movement experience without falling, it shifts their perception to one of the movement is no longer dangerous, and they perceive that they had control over that situation. The more this perception or belief is reinforced through positive movement experiences, the fewer adverse movement strategies are used to avoid falls or pain.[9-12]

A great study by Roller et al[13] looked at a population experiencing fear of falling, and more importantly, a group of individuals who tested as having a "high risk of falls." They found that these participants showed a significant improvement in static and dynamic balance, functional mobility, self-efficacy, and lower extremity active range of motion after a 10-week Pilates intervention consisting of a once-a-week group class. The intervention did not provide any specificity training for fall prevention, merely positive movement experiences that shifted their perception and functional outcomes regarding falling.

In everyday life, we perform a tremendous variety of functional tasks. Each task performed requires an awareness of how the tasks or movements are regulated or constrained.[7] Joseph Pilates said, "Physical fitness is the first requisite of happiness. Our interpretation of physical fitness is the attainment and maintenance of a uniformly developed body with a sound mind, fully capable of naturally, easily, and satisfactorily performing our many and varied daily tasks with spontaneous zest and pleasure."[5] The International Classification of Functioning, Disability and Health tool by the World Health Organization model refers to "participation" as what the individual chooses to participate in, which can greatly affect their ability to move. I regularly see this in my own practice. For example, I had 2 female patients in their late 80s. The first patient was very inactive and was being treated for a shoulder impingement. When I asked her what caused her shoulder pain, she replied, "It only hurts when I am getting my coffee cup down from the second shelf." In my limited wisdom, I asked her what would happen if she placed her coffee cup on the bottom shelf instead. She thought I was a genius, and we discharged her as a happy camper. The second patient had multiple lumbar surgeries, a pacemaker, and a pain modulator implant for her back pain. When I asked her what she believed she should be participating in, she said, "I am an elite golfer and competitive in the senior's division for women." Her choice of participation was much higher than the first patient and required a lot more attention to the tasks that she wanted to successfully perform to be competitive in her sport. These are the types of scenarios in which therapists, teachers, and coaches need to determine what the tasks are that the client wants to perform and what their abilities and limitations are pertaining to those tasks. This is the only way to truly treat or teach the person in front of us. Each client

or patient needs a plan that is specific to their wants and desires. This is where I see our primary purpose as movement practitioners—to assess where the client is and where they want to go and use every possible medium to help them succeed. The Principles of Movement are powerful tools when used to design the pathway toward restoration of functional movement and performance.

Tasks can be influenced by the following factors, which should be taken into consideration when determining the difficulty of the task: discrete vs continuous tasks, stabile vs mobile surfaces, open vs closed tasks, and the complexity level of the task itself. A discrete task has a clear beginning and ending (eg, sit to stand). Once the client is standing, that task is over. Compare this to a continuous activity, such as walking, swimming, or running, where there is no clear start or finish to the task.[14]

The stability and mobility of the surfaces the task is to be performed on can play a large role in the successful execution of the task. Tasks performed with a steady base of support are usually less complex from a task execution standpoint than the same tasks performed while moving. Basketball has both attributes. When shooting a free throw, the feet are planted on the free throw line, and the basketball player shoots the basket. In contrast, when the game is going, the basketball player is often shooting while moving, requiring a lot more coordination (Figures 7-2A and 7-2B). The surface can also be an influencer of the movement execution (eg, skiing on water or snow vs rollerblading on smooth concrete). The snow and water introduce many more challenging variables to the mover than the smooth concrete. However, if I had to fall, I would take the water and snow any day over the concrete.

An open task relates to movements that are not predictable, which are usually determined by the environment (eg, a basketball player does not know ahead of time where the opponent is going to block them and must react based on the movement of the opponent; Figure 7-3). The opposite is true for a

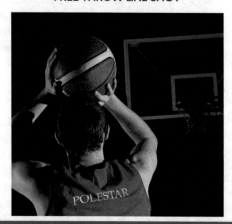

[A]
FREE THROW LINE SHOT

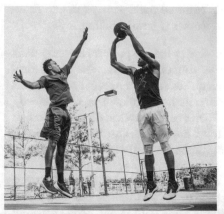

[B]
JUMP SHOT

Figure 7-2. (A) Basketball player at the free throw line. (B) Basketball player shooting with a defender.

(ESB Professional/Shutterstock.com.)

(oneinchpunch/Shutterstock.com.)

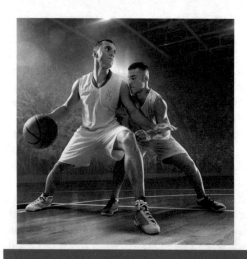

Figure 7-3. Basketball player avoiding a block or steal.

(Alex Kravtsov/Shutterstock.com.)

closed task. For example, a sprinter running a 100-m race has minimal variations and disruptions because the track is a relatively fixed environment.[7,14]

Lastly, the attention continuum influences the complexity of the task. A gross motor activity such as a squat or a lift requires a relatively basic level of attention compared with a fine motor task such as playing a musical instrument or painting in which fine articulation of the hands and fingers are required.

The third major influencer of the organization of movement is the environment. The environment can enhance or impair the movement. There have been many behavioral science studies looking at the environment of where people work. What is the lighting like? It is easier to work efficiently in a well-lit area compared with a dark and undefined office. The temperature, noise, proximity to the toilets or parking area, and relationships with their bosses and coworkers can all have an impact on performance.[15] Other examples of variability include factors such as weather, team sport, noise, and temperature variance, which can challenge the task. The more stable the environment, the less variability and the easier it is to perform the task.

MOTOR THEORY

Motor theory provides a lot of insight into the evolution of motor control science. I have included an evolution, as well as an eclectic composition, of motor theories from the late 1800s to modern times. I find it interesting how the theories do not cancel each other out as much as they continue to build on each other. We are very complex animals, and the factors that influence our movement and learning can be intriguing and diverse.

The reflex theory represents some of the original thoughts of how we as humans acquire and execute movement. Sherrington[16] wrote that reflexes were the building blocks of complex behavior. The simple reflexes are combined into greater actions that wholly constitute the behavior of the individual. His theory was unchallenged for more than 50 years. What we now know is that reflexes cannot account for voluntary movements that occur without a sensory stimulus. The reflex theory cannot explain fast movement such as running, and probably most importantly, it does not explain novel or new movements.[7]

The hierarchical theory proposes that all movement is organized from top down (ie, from the motor cortex and spinal cord levels of function). This did not discredit the reflex theory; rather, it is built on it. Reflexes belong to the lower-level nervous system, and when the higher centers are intact, they will override the reflex control. This can be observed in child growth and development, as well as in neurologic pathologies, such as brain trauma. When injury occurs to a higher center of the nervous system and it no longer functions, the lower reflexes (eg, spasticity) can dominate. An interesting phenomenon known as a *central pattern generator* has been observed in human and animal studies in which a lesion to the central nervous system above a certain level in the spinal cord prevents a voluntary motor pattern, such as taking a step. However, when placed on a treadmill, the reflexive gait pattern in the lower spinal cord allows the individual to walk. This resulted in what is known as

the *reflex/hierarchical theory of motor control.*[7] Current research demonstrates that any part of the human nervous system can act on other levels depending on the tasks.

The motor programming theory advocates that all movement is a result of movement programs built into the central nervous system; it looks at actions rather than reactions. Although this theory is more flexible than the reflex and hierarchical theories, it still has weaknesses. Its assumptions of central pattern generators were apparent in animal science models. In one model, cats were spinalized (ie, the spinal cord was severed [humanely I am sure]) and were still able to walk on a treadmill, showing the motor program existed in the spinal cord below the lesion.[17] The limitation in this model is that it did not take into account other factors that influence movement including the musculoskeletal system and environmental variables in achieving the control of movement when the environment changed.[7]

The systems theory was first introduced by Russian scientist Nikolai Bernstein in the 1920s. Bernstein was looking at the nervous system and body in a different way than the motor plan or hierarchical theories. He realized the nervous system was dependent on the internal and external forces acting on the body. Bernstein was best known for his theory on controlling degrees of freedom. In the process of learning movement, an infant will start with movements requiring limited degrees of freedom. The child then progresses with more complex movements that have increasing degrees of freedom and use more joints and muscles to coordinate to execute the desired task.[8] The systems theory predicted movement behavior much better than previous theories but was limited in its explanation of the interaction of the organism with the environment.[7] Bernstein's theory proved to be beneficial to movement practitioners in that it brought awareness to the fact that movement is not determined solely by the central nervous system but rather by the output of the central nervous system through a mechanical system (ie, our bodies). Bernstein showed that comorbidities such as muscle contractures around the knee or elbow after a neurologic accident to the central nervous system would directly affect the central nervous system's ability to execute a movement pattern. This was a breakthrough regarding the complexity of how our peripheral feedback, whether it is internal or external feedback, can directly impact the ability for the central nervous system to execute a movement.

The dynamic action theory is an exciting theory that resembles the chaos theory. How does order take place in animal movement? How does movement become natural and spontaneous? How do patterns and organization we see in the world come into being from their constituent parts? How do we reduce a system with thousands of degrees of freedom into a system of a few degrees of freedom so we can function naturally and cohesively? We can answer these questions by looking at the principle of self-organization, which is a fundamental dynamic systems principle.[7] It states that when a system of individual parts comes together, its elements behave collectively in an ordered way. There is no need for a higher center issuing instruction or commands to achieve coordinated action. This principle applied to motor control predicts that movement can emerge as a result of interacting elements without the need for specific commands or motor programs from the nervous system.[7] One of the things I find most interesting and applicable to the teaching of movement is that in the dynamic action theory the central nervous system is de-emphasized in the controlling of movement and seeks physical explanations that may contribute to the movement characteristics.[18] The dynamic action theory advocates the effect of attractor wells pertaining to movement. An attractor well can be defined as a visual representation of how a practiced pattern of movement gets ingrained deeper and deeper until something changes to shift the pattern out of its well. For example, when a horse is walking and starts to move faster, at a certain point the movement strategy is no longer efficient, and the horse will shift into a different attractor well, such as trotting. The horse then trots at a faster rate to the point that it is no longer efficient and

moves into a different movement pattern, such as galloping, and so forth. It is thought that the energy expenditure determines the motor program for locomotion. The deeper the attractor well, the more stable and difficult it is to shift into the next well. In contrast, the shallower the well, the less stable and easier it is to shift attractor wells. Of late, the dynamic action theory has adapted many of the principles in the systems theory into a dynamic systems model.[18] According to Shumway-Cook and Woollacott,[7] a limitation in the model can be the presumption that the nervous system has a fairly unimportant role and the relationship between the physical system of the animal and the environment in which it operates primarily determines the animal's behavior. As a therapist, I find this very aspect the most exciting. As important and intriguing as the nervous system is, I do not have to be a brain surgeon or neurologist to understand that movement is largely influenced by the environment (load), the body (mobility, control, and alignment), and the motivation (perception and belief) to execute daily tasks. In my experience, we can greatly influence our clients' ability to experience successful movement and overcome faulty movement patterns by influencing mobility, alignment, control, load, and perception. I had a patient who was recovering from a fractured tibial plateau after a fall. At first, her gait was belabored and painful; her eyes were fixed on the ground in front of her, and her body was hunched over, grabbing everything she could to make sure she was safe. Over the next couple of weeks, we specifically worked on axial alignment, ensuring full extension of the affected knee, and I modified the load to a point that she could tolerate walking without pain. We implemented walking sticks to keep her upright rather than using a walker. The assistance that decreased the external load and a focus on increasing gait tempo resulted in decreased ground reaction force and surface contact time. By the end of the 3 weeks, she was walking with no assistance, with a vertical posture, and at a much faster pace. She commented, "I cannot believe walking faster hurts so much less."

BOX 7-1: EXPERIMENT—ENERGY EXPENDITURE

Pretend that you are walking on a treadmill, and the speed is increased to about 5 to 6 mph/8 to 10 kph; suddenly, you find that you can no longer walk efficiently, and it is now much easier for you to run. You move into a different movement strategy or attractor well. If you bring the speed closer to 9 mph/14 kph, you will find yourself running more on the balls of your feet and sprinting. Then, when you get tired, you will slow the treadmill back to 2 to 3 mph/3 to 4 kph. This will reduce your energy level by reducing the power demand. We know that things like energy expenditure are important. Gravity, load, and length of levers are all things that contribute as influencers of movement.

Lastly, the ecological theory, independent of other motor control theories, researched how the motor systems interact with the environment and goal-oriented behavior.[19] Gibson[19] stated that it was not sensation per se but rather perception that was important to the animal, especially the perception of the environmental factors specifically important to the task. The ecological theory has broadened our thinking of understanding the nervous system from being a sensory-motor system reacting to environment variables to that of a perception-action system that actively explores the environment to satisfy its own goals.[7]

One of the other major influencing factors discussed is perception. We know that our desires, perceptions, fears, and motivations have much more to do with the quality of movement or the movement patterns selected by the motor control systems (ie, muscles, bones, tendons).

A fun example of how motivation affects outcome can be demonstrated by the following situation. Let us imagine that you and I both had to run 5 miles right now. At the end of your 5 miles is a check for $5000 in your name. At the end of my 5 miles is my checkbook so that I can write a check for $5000 to you. Can you imagine how our motivation to run those 5 miles might be different? To you $5000 might be so valuable that you would just run out of the house without shoes or socks. You would not care what surface you were on; you would run those 5 miles and grab your $5000 check. On the other hand, for me, $5000 is a lot of money. If I must write a check to you for $5000 at the end of the 5 miles, I will take my time putting on my shoes. I will probably find some other activities to do that I find are more important. I might get lost. I might walk backwards. I might walk slowly. I might start experiencing pain in my knee, hip, or back because I am not motivated. I have a negative motivation to pay you $5000.

We also know that secondary gains can affect movement and movement strategies (eg, being victimized, being in a car accident, being injured at work). These factors influence how we move or do not move. As therapists and movement educators, we will never understand all the factors that influence movement even if we study them every day of our lives. I want us to understand that there are many factors that influence movement. Do not be closed-minded and think that it is just about a muscle contraction or a joint. As we deal with human beings and teach them to move and to have positive movement experiences, we must take into consideration all the possible factors that can influence successful movement. As we move into the next part of the chapter, it is imperative that we keep an open mind as to how we use this knowledge and these tools to facilitate the acquisition of new movement, increase efficiencies of movement, and learn movement that will be sustainable as it pertains to health and performance.

The takeaway from these different motor control theories is that we can safely emphasize task-oriented approaches to facilitate functional outcomes. We can also assume that normal movement emerges as an interaction among many factors including energy expenditure, mobility, environment, and belief. Movement is organized around behavioral goals and is constrained by the environment. These are all tools we can work with to facilitate successful movement experiences for our clients.

MOTOR LEARNING

Motor learning was defined by Anne Shumway-Cook and and Marjorie Woollacott[7] as a study of acquisition and/or modification of movement. This science is the most applicable to what we do as therapists, teachers, and movement coaches because people usually already know how to move. What we want to find out is if they move efficiently and can participate in their desired functional activities. Faulty movement patterns can be related to poor awareness, postural habits, or compensations because of injury and disease. These faulty movement patterns can interfere with clients' ability to perform their many varied daily tasks spontaneously. Let us further explore how we facilitate the acquisition of new movement, and more importantly, modifications of faulty movement. To achieve this, it is important to search for a task solution, or in other words, a successful movement experience that emerges from an interaction between the individual, the task, and the environment as discussed in the Motor Control section. In motor learning, the word "learning" has a more permanent effect on behavior; hence, short-term alterations of behavior are not thought to be learning.[7,14] This becomes very important for the practitioner to understand, whether we are creating short-term behavioral changes or if our clients are experiencing long-term retention of what we facilitate in our sessions. It is also important that we extend the rules of motor learning to imply

it must be built around solving functional tasks in specific environments.[7] The point I want to make here is if the client is not deeply involved with their learning process through problem-solving and awareness training, it is likely that the outcomes will be more of a short-term change rather than a long-term behavioral change.

Once we take the challenge to facilitate long-term change in our clients, it becomes even more important not to lose sight of other variables that can impact motor learning and performance. Some of these factors include muscle skeletal restrictions, environmental influences, perception, fatigue, anxiety, and motivation. A basic assumption is to try and eliminate as many of these factors as possible to optimize motor learning.

There are many forms of learning that have been extensively studied in human and animal research. Two common motor learning concepts are discussed: nonassociative and associative learning.

Nonassociative learning forms are based on a single stimulus that can either habituate a response to that stimulus by decreasing the responsiveness to the stimulus or can sensitize the response to the stimulus by increasing the sensitivity to the stimulus. I use habituation quite often with my patients who suffer from hypersensitivity. The repeated stimulus at graded levels can decrease their sensitivity to a more normal threshold, allowing them to function better. It is also used quite often with dizziness and used to decrease the sensitivity to motion.

Sensitization is also useful and can be used to increase a client's sensitivity to spatial orientations. An example of sensitization is a person who has suffered from a stroke and experiences neglect on one side. The therapist can use a repeated stimulus to that side to increase the awareness of the arm in space with an activity such as reaching. The key difference between nonassociative and associative forms of learning is that nonassociative learning has a single repeated stimulus to create a functional outcome. Associative is a higher form of learning and involves making an association, like the word suggests, of ideas.

Associative forms of learning can be categorized as classical conditioning and operant conditioning. A famous experiment involving a classical conditioning model was with Ivan Pavlov's dogs. The outcome was that the dogs salivated when a bell rang. How did this occur? Pavlov associated the sound of a bell with the presentation of food. The dogs were conditioned to connect the idea that when the bell sounded, food was about to be delivered. What do we do when we get ready to eat something delicious? We salivate. Another important fact about classical conditioning is that the association is most effective if the association of ideas is tied into a life-sustaining idea. In Pavlov's dog experiments, it was food. How do we create postural and movement associations with life-sustaining ideas? The reward must be something the client is truly interested in. Then, we must make sure we can provide them with a reward for the behavior after the stimulus until it becomes natural. Several health-based apps are using wearables to create stimuli and rewards for behavioral changes.

Operant conditioning is another form of associative learning that is basically trial-and-error learning. The response is built on a consequence. The principle is that behaviors that are rewarded are repeated even at the cost of other behaviors. The reverse of this is true also. If an adverse stimulus is associated with a behavior, then we are less likely to repeat that behavior. This adverse association interests me because it involves pain, falls, and fear. Negative stimuli (eg, movement equals pain or movement increases my risk of falls) limits the individual's desire to move. This type of learning can be very difficult to unlearn when the rewards or consequences are so strong (eg, fear avoidance). When we can provide a positive movement experience without pain or with increased balance and confidence, the individual is more likely to repeat the new behavior.

From an operant conditioning perspective, we want to make sure that our clients are getting far more positive rewards related to their movement experiences to ensure a healthier movement behavior.

Associative learning can further be classified into 2 categories based on the type and recall of information learned: declarative and procedural learning.[7] This is most relevant and applicable with human motor learning. Declarative learning depends on awareness, attention, and reflection. It also depends on the practitioner first providing external feedback to be able to provide the client with heightened awareness. External feedback consists of verbal and tactile cueing or recording a video of the client and showing it to them. Individuals will respond better to different types of external feedback (ie, vision, auditory, kinesthetic, tactile). At the beginning of the client-practitioner relationship, the practitioner will need to provide the client with more external feedback and encourage the development of internal feedback and reflection. As the relationship continues, the practitioner should spend more time prompting internal feedback and awareness with the following questions: How does that feel to you? What do you notice when you add this to the movement sequence? and How does breathing this way or that way affect the movement? Once they have consciously gained internal awareness through practice, they move into procedural learning. This stage is when the individual must practice, practice, practice, practice, and repeat what they have learned. Procedural learning does not require heightened awareness but rather repetition. This is the first step toward spontaneous and natural movement while performing our many varied daily tasks.[5] Correct practice form is necessary with procedural learning. One can practice bad form repeatedly and end up with a deeply ingrained faulty pattern. Therefore, a home exercise program that is not followed up on by the practitioner might end up with a less than desirable outcome.

MOTOR LEARNING THEORIES

Motor learning theories are like motor control theories; many of the pioneer thinkers and researchers investigated how we as humans learn to move, and more importantly, how we facilitate the recovery of function. Jack A. Adams's closed-loop theory proposed a closed-loop process in which sensory feedback is used for the ongoing production of skilled movement. Much of his theory was built on the reflex theory that sensory feedback was necessary for controlling movement. He believed there were 2 distinct types of movement memory: a memory trace and a perceptual trace. The memory trace is used in the selection and initiation of the movement pattern, whereas the perceptual trace is built up through practice (ie, the more the patient or client practices, the stronger the perceptual trace becomes). He further purported that the accuracy of movement is directly related to the strength of the perceptual trace.[20] A limitation of Adams's theory is its inability to explain the accurate performance of novel movements or movements made in an open loop without sensory feedback. There is research that supports that varied movement practice patterns may improve performance. This is discussed later. What I do appreciate in Adams's theory is the concept of perceptual trace and that practice increases accuracy or the ability to be spontaneous in movement strategies.

The schema theory by Richard A. Schmidt emphasizes open-loop control processes and a generalized motor program concept.[21] His theory implies that the individual learns a general set of rules that can be applied to a variety of contexts. The term *schema* in psychology literature refers to an abstract representation stored in memory. For example, I have a signature that has a look and style. This same signature can be executed with fine motor of my right and dominant hand but can also be done with my left, nondominant hand. It may not be as pretty, but you will see the elements of my signature. To make this more exciting,

I could write my signature on a chalkboard with a completely different motor program, with my foot in the sand, or with my mouth with a paintbrush. The point is that there is an abstract memory of my signature, and it does not matter which part of my body I use to express my signature; traces of the style, look, and feel will be manifested even though the motor program is different for each signature strategy. At the heart of Schmidt's schema is the generalized motor program, which contains the general rules. Schmidt proposed that after an individual makes movement, 4 things are stored in memory: the initial movement conditions, the parameters used in the generalized motor program, knowledge of the results, and sensory consequences (ie, how it looked, sounded, felt). Schmidt also believed that variability of practice should improve motor learning.[21] Further research of Schmidt's theory of variability of practice reported mixed outcomes. Possible factors include the age of the individual learning and previous experiences; if an adult has already learned a movement strategy, it might have less of an effect than on a child who is more naive and possibly has not learned that behavior.[7]

The ecological theory draws on both the systems and the ecological theories of motor control. Newell[22] suggested that motor learning is a process that increases the coordination between perception and action in a way consistent with the task and environmental constraints. The human is always seeking the optimal strategies to solve the task. This involves not only the most appropriate motor response for the task but also the most appropriate perceptual cues as well.[22] Perceptual cues that are critical to how a task is executed are also referred to as *regulatory cues*.[23] Optimal solutions require the optimal regulatory cue and optimal movement strategy for the specific task. This is apparent to me when I am teaching a group class and use a refined and proven verbal cue to facilitate a movement, but 1 or 2 individuals in the class do not respond to the cue or image. I then must resort to finding another image or provide tactile cueing to facilitate the desired movement strategy of the individual(s). Shumway-Cook and Woollacott[7] stated that motor learning is characterized by optimal task-relevant mapping of perception and action and not by a rule-based representation of action. The discovery of optimal strategy and optimal perceptual cues reminds me a lot of what Moshe Feldenkrais discovered in his method of movement acquisition. Allowing the individual the opportunity to discover a strategy to accomplish a task is very powerful, and I believe this is more likely to meet the criteria for motor learning and permanency. When the individual is free from a novel movement being right or wrong, they can feel and reflect through their own senses if that strategy is efficient. It is not a matter of being a bad mover or a good mover, only the constant seeking to be a better mover. I believe that seeking efficiency in all we do is a trait innate in humans. As facilitators of movement, we can guide the movement exploration process more than teaching them what muscle needs to contract first and how much. My experience is that this prescriptive style of teaching is a hopeless way of ever achieving natural and spontaneous motor strategies in people. Animals and infants do not learn this way. An optimal movement strategy does not typically happen all at once and often comes in stages of learning.

The stages of motor learning are thought by some to be a unique theory of motor learning in and of themselves. The human acquires an initial stage of skill and continues to learn over time. In the psychology literature, Fitts and Posner[24] described this happening in 3 stages. In the first stage, the learner is concerned with understanding the nature of the task, which requires a very high level of attention. It is known as the *cognitive stage of learning*. In this stage, the person is experimenting, exploring, and discovering what works and what does not work. You could call it the sampler of movement strategies. As movement facilitators, we are often overbearing when trying to teach clients to move instead of allowing the discovery and giving permission to explore.

Fitts and Posner[24] called the second stage the *associative stage*. By now, the person has selected the best strategy for the task and begins to refine the skill. Schmidt stated that at this stage the person is more interested in refining the skill rather than selecting the best strategy. In stage 2, the person can practice, and this takes time; hopefully, the natural human instinct follows to make it efficient. It is unfortunate in our fitness world that we have confused being ripped and thin with being efficient. The hard body workout does not seem to follow the movement strategy usually used by children and animals. I guess it is more the aesthetic and sex hormones that drive the need for the hard body look. It would have to be something as strong as sex hormones to override the drive to be efficient.

The third stage according to Fitts and Posner is the *autonomous stage*; this stage can be defined by the low amount of attention required for the performance of the task. At this stage, the individual can devote attention to other aspects of the task, such as the environment. This makes me think of soccer players. Learning to handle and dribble the ball begins with the discovery of what is the best way to handle the ball. They watch great soccer players, and they start to learn strategies; they then move into stage 2 where they are practicing their ballhandling skills until they become very efficient but that still does not make them a great soccer player. I have seen many soccer players who are great ballhandlers but are not great soccer players. In stage 3, the ballhandling is second nature, and their attention is now focused on the strategy of the field, the competitor, and, most importantly, the goal (Figure 7-4).

The systems 3-stage model is yet another theory that relates to Bernstein's systems theory of motor control. The emphasis is on controlling the degrees of freedom as a central theme to learning a new movement. Vereijken et al[25] used this approach to develop a model of the stages of motor learning in which the first stage is the *novice stage*; in this stage, the learner simplifies the movement to reduce the

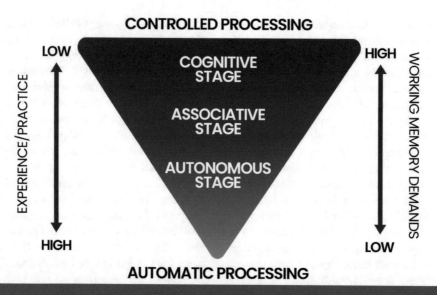

CONTROLLED PROCESSING

COGNITIVE STAGE

ASSOCIATIVE STAGE

AUTONOMOUS STAGE

EXPERIENCE/PRACTICE — LOW / HIGH

WORKING MEMORY DEMANDS — HIGH / LOW

AUTOMATIC PROCESSING

Figure 7-4. Paul Morris Fitts and Michael I. Posner's model for learning.

degrees of freedom. This is done by creating cocontractions at multiple joints to minimize the complexity of the learning. The sacrifice is efficiency and flexibility in adapting to the environment. In this stage, I think of the novice learning to ride a bike for the first time. The body is very rigid, and the bike wobbles a lot, but they learn. The second stage, called the *advanced stage*, is one in which the performer begins to release additional degrees of freedom by allowing movements at more joints involved in the task. This results in a much more efficient and fluid execution of the movement. In this stage, the bicycle rider can now ride the bike with no hands and can control the bike with only their legs, relying on synergies throughout the body to execute efficient movement and stay balanced. The third stage is called the *expert stage*; I call this the *Cirque du Soleil stage*. Very few people ever get to the point where they are efficiently releasing all the thousands of degrees of freedom and spontaneously controlling them. In this stage, the individual has learned to take advantage of the musculoskeletal system and the environment to optimize the efficiency of the movement.[7,25] This 3-stage model has great application to Pilates equipment work and certain forms of

yoga in which props are used to assist or limit the degrees of freedom in the first stage of learning. By providing external support to the person in the early phases of learning a motor skill, we can expedite success by using a graded progression and the appropriate addition of degrees of freedom and the decrease of support. In Polestar, we often refer to this strategy as *creating a positive movement experience*. We can manipulate gravity, the length of levers, assistance, the number of joints involved, and alignment to create an optimal learning environment, especially for patients with more severe neurologic impairments. The goal often is to create an environment that can be associated by the patient or client with a functional task (eg, rolling, bed mobility, sit to stand, stairs, walking).

Gentile[23] proposed a 2-stage model. In the first stage, the goal of the learner is to develop an understanding of the task dynamics; this includes discovering the strategy and exploring the effect of the environment on the task. In this stage, the learner is discovering what is relevant and what is not relevant. I really appreciate this stage when teaching. So often teachers vomit hundreds of verbal cues and images to the client, and the truth is they cannot process it, let alone discover what is and what is not important. One of the most disruptive external cues is a muscle contraction (eg, "Squeeze your glutes," "Pull your belly to your spine," or "Lift your pelvic floor"). I believe that the client needs the time to make sense of the movement, and it might not happen in the first few attempts. Once they do figure it out, they progress into the second stage called the *fixation/diversification stage*. This refers to open vs closed skills in which the person is developing the ability to adapt and improve consistency and efficiency. Performing the task in a nonpredictable environment is practiced at this level. An example of this is the basketball player who has learned proper shooting mechanics and is now challenged in stage 2 by having to be guarded by an opponent or dribble with both hands to avoid someone stealing the ball from them. This again requires movement diversification and spontaneous reactions.[7,23]

In Polestar, we use another model with 4 stages with the intention of achieving unconscious competence (Figure 7-5). It is thought that this model was developed by a business coach named Noel Burch in 1970 for Gordon Training International. Stage 1 is *unconscious incompetence*. This is when a novice does not have any awareness of the desired movement strategy they are about to learn; basically, they don't know what they don't know. Poor postural awareness could fit into this stage (eg, the person is not aware of their slouched posture and how it is affecting their locomotion). Stage 2, *conscious incompetence*, is when the person is now aware of the incompetence in their movement either through their senses (internal feedback) or externally from pictures, video, or their teacher. We do not want to spend much time in this state; it is neither productive nor positive for the person. Stage 3, *conscious competence*, could be the progression from declarative learning to procedural learning in which the movement becomes natural, efficient, and spontaneous, which leads to

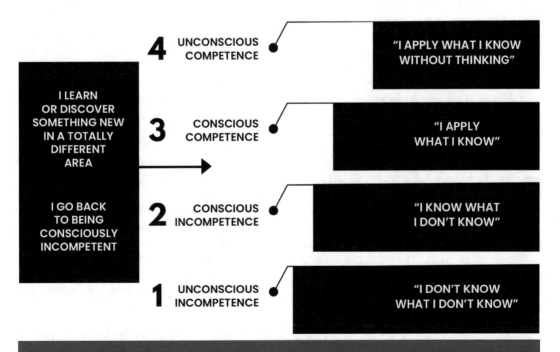

Figure 7-5. Four stages to achieve unconscious competence.

stage 4, *unconscious competence* (see Figure 7-5). This is what Joseph Pilates referred to when discussing how we perform our daily activities spontaneously with vigor and zest.[5]

> **"PHYSICAL FITNESS IS THE FIRST REQUISITE OF HAPPINESS."**
> **—JOSEPH PILATES[5]**

APPLICATIONS AND SKILLS

I want to explore how we can use different forms of feedback to deepen our patients' and clients' understanding of movement. Extrinsic vs intrinsic feedback, how much feedback is enough, and what is the difference between internal and external feedback are questions that often arise when teaching movement. Internal feedback is the information that comes to the individual simply through the various sensory systems in the body. This includes visual, proprioception, touch, pressure, auditory, and even smell and taste. This is how someone might know their arm is up even if their eyes are closed. In some cases and in particular parts of the body, awareness is quite low and might require external feedback to calibrate with the intrinsic feedback systems. Extrinsic feedback often complements intrinsic feedback. It can come from cameras, electromyography, biofeedback, instruction, images, tactile cueing, and corrective positioning. Extrinsic feedback can be delivered in 2 forms, concurrently with the task or after the task, which is known as *terminal feedback*. Masterful cueing is a powerful tool for the practitioner. Learning how much is too much and how much is not enough can only be accomplished through experience. Just like our clients learn to move through trial and error so do we when learning to cue. The variables and obstacles that make each learning experience unique also make each teaching experience unique. Masterful teaching is a higher-level skill and requires awareness of how clients respond to cueing and instruction. We should ask ourselves what some of the obstacles or unique variables are with our different clients. This information will shift how we provide extrinsic feedback. Ideally, we want to create as many opportunities as possible for the client to experience intrinsic feedback and be more of a compass for the client so that what they are feeling correlates with the task at hand.

Understanding the rules of practice is another very powerful skill for the practitioner to use to help create optimal learning experiences for the client. I have studied this skill for years and am still discovering pearls of wisdom on how I can do a better job of creating optimal learning environments for our clients. The assumption that a client or patient would simply go home and practice the exercises that were on a sheet of paper we handed them has proven to be overrated and poorly effective in achieving successful outcomes.[26] Variables such as fatigue, understanding, anxiety, distraction, and motivation are all viable factors that influence the success of our clients' practice. It helps to understand human behavior when it comes to motivation to practice.

Constant vs variable feedback pertains to whether the tasks that we are teaching will be ones needed to be performed in a relatively constant, predictable environment or an adverse environment at different tempos or with other obstacles that require spontaneous adaptability. For example, let us choose walking as the task. If someone's goal is to efficiently walk on a treadmill at 4 mph, then constant practice on the treadmill will result in the most productive outcome. However, if you want to walk on a busy street in New York or must cover icy terrain, it would be much more efficacious to practice in conditions that vary and are related to the goal. The closer you can practice in the environment in which the client will have to participate, the better their results will be.

Random vs blocked feedback is another way of practicing and warrants discussion. A blocked practice is to repeat the same task repeatedly, then move on to the subsequent task and practice it, and then move on to the next task. Let us say there are 5 sub-tasks required to stand up from a chair. In blocked practice, we would first work on moving the feet under the chair multiple times; the next block would be scooting the bottom forward and back on the chair. You get the idea. Random practice would be practicing all the subtasks in sequence. There is evidence that the more difficult the practice, the better the outcome of performing the task is; it may be slower, but the long-term retention of the movement task is better.[14]

Whole vs part feedback and training are controversial. The conversation is around breaking the task down into small parts for training and if that in turn will facilitate a whole functional movement pattern. I am particularly interested in this whole form of practice. Evidence continues to show that training the whole is better than parts and that isolated training (eg, training of a quadricep) has little to no carryover when standing or walking unless the client can make the connection. This can be observed in core control training. Research indicated that people with low back pain showed poor motor control of the abdominal wall, especially the transverse abdominis (TA).[27,28] We hypothesized that if we strengthened the TA, it would restore normal motor control to the core muscles, and the back pain would disappear.[27] What we have learned over the years is that the TA works subconsciously and subthreshold, meaning that an isolated contraction of the TA probably will not carry over to a normal load response of the trunk musculature with daily tasks.[27,29-32] For it to work correctly, it would need to be trained according to the desired task (eg, stand up without back pain). How do we re-educate the TA in a simple activity, such as sit to stand? If we tell someone to engage the muscle or perform a volitional contraction, then we have not successfully cued all the different muscle actions that lead to function and most likely will not have a desirable outcome. This raises the following question: How well does isolated training transfer into functional tasks? Research would lead us to believe that specificity training is the best, but I have also seen how

whole body training has surpassed isolated or block training. Increasing the opportunity for the client to discover the most efficient strategy pertaining to their desired task seems to have the best outcome.

Variables pertaining to memory and cognitive impairments can be a large obstacle in learning new movement. This can be seen when working with clients who experience dementia or poor physical awareness because of Parkinson disease. It is necessary to be patient and only work as much as the client's cognitive capacity tolerates in that session. You might also discover with some memory and cognitive impairments that there are better times of the day to train. For clients with Parkinson disease, medication can also affect cognition and alertness during a session. Find out when the best time to work is and schedule sessions accordingly. By using tools such as alignment, load, and tempo as they pertain to the many varied daily tasks of our clients, we can provide the discovery, awareness, and efficiency we seek in motor learning and functional outcomes.

BIOENERGETICS

There is a growing body of research discussing gene expression changes induced by mind-body work.[33] A recent systematic review of 18 relevant studies showed that there was a reversed genetic expression often associated with chronic stress and inflammatory diseases after practicing mind-body interventions.[34] I am sure that we are going to see a growing body of knowledge and science demonstrating how mind-body interventions influence change in human physiology.

The anecdotal stories of positive changes are endless for those who practice mind-body modalities; I have certainly experienced many myself. In my travels teaching Pilates and physical therapy, I still have people come up to me and say, "I love what you talk about with the body, but I do not see where the mind and the spirit have any relationship to movement and health." I refer them back to Joseph Pilates' guiding principles in which he stated the following: "Whole body health is about the uniform development of the body, the mind, and the spirit."[5] You cannot separate them. Even if you choose to say, "I do not want to have anything to do with the mind or the spirit," you are still influencing it. I want to share this idea with you. A balanced movement throughout the entire system supports a balanced flow of energy throughout all energetic systems. When I first learned Pilates in 1987, there was no program or school. We would go observe the masters and come back home and practice. As mentioned in earlier chapters, one of the practice habits that I incorporated early on was to go through all the exercises as a different system in my body, including the skeletal, muscular, nervous, integumentary, digestive, respiratory, circulatory, and lymphatic systems. I would go through the movement focusing on how the Pilates movement affected all the systems of my body. It took me about 2 years. That is when I started gaining an appreciation of how movement affects my digestion, circulation, and other systems in my body. People who do Pilates often say afterward, "I am having more regular bowel movements since starting Pilates or yoga." People call me and say, "I could not get pregnant before and now I am pregnant." They have also commented on how their blood pressure has normalized and that the swelling in their feet and ankles has diminished. Granted, these are anecdotal, but we see and hear them all the time from our clients who regularly perform their Pilates, yoga, and Gyrotonic Expansion System exercises. Over the last several years, I have also had the chance to learn more about bioenergetics, particularly the myofascial system, acupuncture, and Ayurvedic medicine. What I realized is that as we move the body, we are moving all the systems of our body, including our bioenergetic system (ie, qi/prana/light/spirit or whatever you choose to call it). It is amazing to me to observe the energetic change in people who have practiced and incorporated these mindful movement practices into their lifestyle. They have energy exuding from their bodies. You can see the light around them, and you can feel their energy. It flows out of everything they say and everything they do. I think this is what Joseph Pilates was referring to when he said "to maximize our potential." We are not just teaching people exercises. I cringe when I hear these different movement practices referred to only as core control exercises or that they are great for toning up your abs and triceps. Although those are common positive outcomes, there are much deeper benefits to discover. The most powerful tool these movement methods provide for us is an increased awareness of ourselves. I believe that as we increase awareness of ourselves through movement, we increase awareness of how our actions influence others in our circles. The more individuals with an increased awareness of self, the closer we get to the critical mass necessary for a peaceful world. I am comfortable saying, even though I do not have evidence, that mindful people do not feel like stealing, harming others, lying, or cheating after a Gyrotonic Expansion System, yoga, Feldenkrais Method, or Pilates class. I have observed an increase in kindness, compassion for others, and volunteerism; a decrease in self-centered beliefs; and overall happier individuals who practice mindful movement. As Joseph Pilates said, the first requisite for happiness is a uniformly developed body, mind, and spirit; fully capable of performing their many varied daily tasks, naturally, easily with spontaneous vigor and zest.[5] Be happy!

OPEN-ENDED QUESTIONS

1 Give an example of how you might integrate all the movement principles to improve your client's movement. How might you prioritize which principle receives greater weight?

2 Define in your own words how a "positive movement experience without pain or that exceeds expectations" might influence ability, perception of well-being, and happiness. How can this influence one's participation according to the International Classification of Functioning, Disability and Health model?

3 Define motor control. Discuss how the many degrees of freedom in human actions are controlled. How does this differ from the definition of human movement? Explain in your own words.

4 Describe the senses that influence perception. How does the integration of sensory impressions have meaning psychologically? Give an example of how something you have smelled, seen, or felt influenced your movement.

5 What must happen for cognition to be effective in the way we execute movement? Explain how your cognition can influence the attention, motivation, and emotional aspects of motor control.

6 How does perception and cognition influence the ability to take action? Where do these patterns of movement exist?

7 How might perception, cognition, and action affect someone's ability to learn after experiencing a very painful experience? Using the same experience, how can you use awareness, thought, and action to create a successful outcome?

8 How might an individual's belief of what they want or should be able to participate in influence their functional outcomes? How might you change your focus to align with their beliefs?

9 Describe in your own words how discrete and continuous tasks differ in terms of the complexity of the movements. Give examples of each. Do the same for open and closed tasks.

10 Give examples of environmental factors that can influence human movement performance. How might you improve the environment of a client or patient you are working with?

11 Give a brief description of each of the following motor theories. What is the premise for each?
   a. Reflexive theory
   b. Hierarchical theory
   c. Motor programming theory
   d. Systems theory
   e. Dynamical action theory
   f. Ecological theory

OPEN-ENDED QUESTIONS

12 Express your own takeaways of how the motor theories can help you understand and apply motor learning. Which one resonates best with you as a movement teacher? Can you see how you can use all in the process of adapting or learning new movement?

13 Define motor learning in your own words. How might this be more applicable to teachers of movement or therapists than the theories of motor control?

14 Why should an individual be deeply engaged in their learning process? What are the likely consequences of teaching movement to an individual who has not engaged in the learning process? How might this affect functional outcomes and independence in activities of daily living?

15 Give examples of nonassociative learning that include habituation and sensitization. How might you use either one to achieve a positive outcome in movement acquisition?

16 Explain in your own words the difference between classical and operant conditioning. How might we use associative learning to benefit or improve movement outcomes?

17 As it pertains to managing clients with chronic pain, how might you use operant conditioning to minimize the learned guarding effects of pain and loss of function? What would become the overarching goal of the treatment or intervention?

18 Create an example of declarative learning and procedural learning of a familiar task. Which would you begin the movement lesson with to optimize awareness? How do you make it subconscious and spontaneous movement?

19 Give a brief description of each of the following motor learning theories. What is the premise for each? What are the strengths and weaknesses of each?
   a. Closed-loop theory
   b. Schema theory
   c. Ecological theory
   d. Stages of motor learning
   e. Systems 3-stage model
   f. 2-stage model
   g. Stages of competence model

20 Give a brief description of each of the following practice applications to optimize learning. What is the premise for each?
   a. Extrinsic vs intrinsic feedback
   b. Rules of practice
   c. Constant vs variable feedback
   d. Random vs blocked feedback
   e. Whole vs part feedback

21 Give an example of how successful movement experiences have changed an emotion or belief you have held. How would you explain an anecdotal statement from a client who, after working with you, says, "I am HAPPIER"?

REFERENCES

1. Strom D. *Coaching and consulting.* 2017; www.dawn-strom.com

2. Cohen BB. *Sensing, Feeling, and Action The Experiential Anatomy of Body-Mind Centering.* 6th ed. Contact Editors; 1993.

3. Singer MA. *The Untethered Soul: The Journey Beyond Yourself.* New Harbinger Publications; 2007.

4. Maslow AH. *Motivation and Personality.* Pearson Education; 1997.

5. Pilates JH, Robbins J, Van Heuit-Robbins L. *Pilates Evolution: The 21st Century.* Presentation Dynamics; 2012.

6. Pilates JH. *Return to Life Through Contrology.* J. J. Augustin Publisher; 1945.

7. Shumway-Cook A, Woollacott MH. *Motor Control Theory and Practical Applications.* 2nd ed. Lippincott Williams & Wilkins; 2001.

8. Bernstein N. *The Coordination and Regulation of Movement.* Pergamon; 1967.

9. Anderson BD. *Randomized Clinical Trial Comparing Active Versus Passive Approaches to the Treatment of Recurrent and Chronic Low Back Pain* [dissertation]. University of Miami; 2005.

10. Mannion AF, Junge A, Taimela S, Muntener M, Lorenzo K, Dvorak J. Active therapy for chronic low back pain: part 3. Factors influencing self-rated disability and its change following therapy. *Spine (Phila Pa 1976).* 2001;26(8):920-929.

11. Mannion AF, Taimela S, Muntener M, Dvorak J. Active therapy for chronic low back pain part 1. Effects on back muscle activation, fatigability, and strength. *Spine (Phila Pa 1976).* 2001;26(8):897-908.

12. Lackner JM, Carosella AM. The relative influence of perceived pain control, anxiety, and functional self efficacy on spinal function among patients with chronic low back pain. *Spine (Phila Pa 1976).* 1999;24(21):2254-2260; discussion 2260-2251.

13. Roller M, Kachingwe A, Beling J, Ickes D-M, Cabot A, Shrier G. Pilates reformer exercises for fall risk reduction in older adults: a randomized controlled trial. *J Bodyw Mov Ther.* 2018;22(4):983-998.

14. Schmidt R. *Motor Control and Learning.* 2nd ed. Human Kinetics; 1988.

15. Lamb S, Kwok KCS. A longitudinal investigation of work environment stressors on the performance and wellbeing of office workers. *Appl Ergon.* 2016;52:104-111.

16. Sherrington CS. *The Integrative Action of the Nervous System.* 2nd ed. Yale University; 1947.

17. Martinez M, Rossignol S. A dual spinal cord lesion paradigm to study spinal locomotor plasticity in the cat. *Ann N Y Acad Sci.* 2013;1279:127-134. doi: 10.1111/j.1749-6632.2012.06823.x

18. Perry S. Clinical implications of a dynamical systems theory. *Neurol Rep.* 1998;22:4-10.

19. Gibson J. *The Senses Considered as Perceptual Systems.* Houghton Mifflin; 1966.

20. Adams JA. A closed-loop theory of motor learning. *J Mot Behav.* 1971;3:111-150.

21. Schmidt R. A schema theory of discrete motor skill learning. *Psychol Rev.* 1975;82:225-260.

22. Newell K. Motor skill acquisition. *Annu Rev Psychol.* 1991;42:213-237.

23. Gentile A. The nature of skill acquisition: therapeutic implications for children with movement disorders. In: Forssberg H, Hirschfield H, eds. *Movement Disorders in Children.* Karger; 1992:31-40.

24. Fitts PM, Posner MI. *Human Performance.* Brooks/Cole; 1967.

25. Vereijken B, van Emmerik REA, Whiting HTA, Newell KM. Freezing degrees of freedom in skill acquisition. *J Mot Behav.* 1992;24:133-142.

26. Anar SÖ. The effectiveness of home-based exercise programs for low back pain patients. *J Phys Ther Sci.* 2016;28(10):2727-2730.

27. Hodges PW, Richardson CA. Inefficient muscular stabilization of the lumbar spine associated with low back pain: a motor control evaluation of transversus abdominis. *Spine (Phila Pa 1976).* 1996;21(22):2640-2650.

28. Lederman E. The fall of the postural-structural-biomechanical model in manual and physical therapies: exemplified by lower back pain. *J Bodyw Mov Ther.* 2011;15(2):131-138.

29. McGill S. *Low Back Disorders: Evidence-Based Prevention and Rehabilitation.* 2nd ed. Human Kinetics; 2007.

30. Richardson C. *Therapeutic Exercise for Spinal Segmental Stabilization in Low Back Pain: Scientific Basis and Clinical Approach.* Churchill Livingstone; 1999.

31. Richardson C, Hodges PW, Hides J. *Therapeutic Exercise for Lumbopelvic Stabilization: A Motor Control Approach for the Treatment and Prevention of Low Back Pain.* 2nd ed. Churchill Livingstone; 2004.

32. Tsao H, Hodges PW. Immediate changes in feed-forward postural adjustments following voluntary motor training. *Exp Brain Res.* 2007;181(4):537-546.

33. Buric I, Farias M, Jong J, Mee C, Brazil IA. What is the molecular signature of mind-body interventions? A systematic review of gene expression changes induced by meditation and related practices. *Front Immunol.* 2017;8:670.

34. Cahn BR, Goodman MS, Peterson CT, Maturi R, Mills PJ. Yoga, meditation and mind-body health: increased BDNF, cortisol awakening response, and altered inflammatory marker expression after a 3-month yoga and meditation retreat. *Front Hum Neurosci.* 2017;11:315.

APPLICATIONS OF THE PRINCIPLES OF MOVEMENT AND CONCLUSION

THE 5 PRINCIPLES OF MOVEMENT SHOULD BE USED TO ASSESS CURRENT CAPACITY AND LIMITATIONS AND TO DEVELOP DYNAMIC MOVEMENT INTERVENTIONS TO ACHIEVE THE INDIVIDUAL'S GOALS.

CHAPTER 8

KEY TERMS
- Biological plasticity
- Graded load
- Human phenotypes
- International Classification of Functioning, Disability and Health
- Perception
- Polestar Assessment Tool
- Principles of Movement
- Qualitative movement

Research in the field of movement science continues to expand, discovering additional variables and factors that influence movement and how movement impacts happiness and health. The trend is leaning heavily toward heightened consciousness and feedback-based exercise regimens that seem to positively influence belief, perception of ability, and well-being. These 5 Principles of Movement are designed to help the practitioner assess what activities their client believes they should be participating in and what the individual's current capacity is to participate or not in the desired activities, and then develop a dynamic intervention to achieve these goals. I have mentioned multiple times within this text that I believe when we can improve our spatial awareness, we improve the alignment between the perception and belief of our body and its reality. This paradigm shift of perception toward reality greatly heightens our consciousness of how intertwined humans are physically, mentally, emotionally, and spiritually. This is especially powerful when approached from a nonsensationalizing or catastrophizing lens. When the practitioner helps the client to identify what they can do and how to successfully move at a level at which they believe they should be able to move, something changes in the psyche of the client. Pain decreases, function increases, hope increases, and most importantly, there is a shift in contentment and happiness. This is the makings for the next book.

Anderson BD.
Principles of Movement (pp 172–196).
© 2024 Taylor & Francis Group.

Science is really moving in a great direction. Those of us who are interested in movement science, especially as it pertains to working with pathologies, have much to learn as science and research evolve. In June 2019, a compilation of articles came out in the *Journal of Orthopaedic & Sports Physical Therapy* reflecting on the role of motor control in low back pain. It was one of the best-written commentaries I have read, and I was impressed with the many factors that influence how humans move. Influencers of human movement can include phenotypes of patients' strategies, how they adapt when they are experiencing low back pain,[1,2] and the fact that there are many unique characteristics of how individuals respond to load.[1-10] Van Dieën et al[10] summarized how even though we need more research, the trend will continue to move toward the individualization of exercise programs built around motor learning styles. More complicated concepts were introduced by Paul Hodges regarding biological plasticity and low back pain and how there are biological adaptations that seem to be affected by painful experiences, especially as they relate to the sensorimotor aspects of the central nervous system.[5,6,9] This results in the creation of diverse interpretations of the nociceptor activity individual by individual. As we better understand the diversity in pain interpretation, neuromuscular responses, historical perspective of pain in the individual, and physiological and psychological adaptation, we can start to see how complex and beautiful movement science is. Qualitative and conscious movement training will continue to become a big part of the future of motor learning, especially in therapeutic interventions. By enhancing awareness and being able to improve our use of external and internal feedback tools, we can improve the alignment between perception and reality. I use the word reality in a framework to understand what the real needs of the client are, not a fabricated one that is applied in a blanket strategy. How do we discover the individual in front of us and truly understand their needs from a movement practitioner's perspective?

Perception continues to be a growing focus of research, especially how it influences a change in behavior. Perception is a powerful predictor of the client's prognosis. The question for us should be the following: How will we choose to influence our client's belief system? Will it be through creating positive movement experiences without pain? Will it be through graded load exercises that progress toward a more functional load desired by the client? Will it be through a restoration of mobility that alleviates stress in other parts of the body and allows pain-free movement? Will it be through regaining motor control of the body through meaningful external and internal feedback strategies, including imagery, tactile and verbal cueing, and internal reflection? All the tools in this book, if used with the right intention, can be strong influencers of change.

It is my desire that the Principles of Movement is used by all movement practitioners to enhance their skill set in terms of the qualitative aspects of movement and the power that comes through sound motor learning science. As we become competent in our understanding of the Principles of Movement, we can then leverage them to help us with the assessment, prescription, and prediction of outcomes. A standardized model, the ICF, can be incorporated to enhance the client's outcome.

INTERNATIONAL CLASSIFICATION OF FUNCTIONING, DISABILITY AND HEALTH MODEL

The World Health Organization developed the ICF.[11] The overall aim of the ICF model is to provide a unified, standard language and framework for the description of health and health-related states. The ICF model allows for a more holistic classification of the individual's health (Figure 8-1). The key words that I want us to focus on in this section are "participation" and "activity." If these become the central focus of our assessments and program designs, the measurable outcomes will greatly improve.

The ICF model includes the following components:

- **Participation:** This pertains to the individual's lifestyle, including work, recreation, family, and community. The type of employment can determine the participation restrictions. If an individual's job consists of heavy labor, a small strain might result in the inability to participate in work-related activities, whereas a similar injury for a sedentary job might have much fewer limitations. This can also apply to activities of daily living, from personal hygiene to community locomotion and/ or more advanced participation found in recreational activities. Participation is often dependent on the individual's expectation of lifestyle, including activities of daily living, work-related activities, and recreation.

- **Activity:** Limitations in performing certain motions or maintaining certain postures or positions are common in people suffering from low back pain. These limitations, as they pertain to low back pain, include walking, running, squatting, lifting, prolonged sitting, standing, and repetitive movements like bending, reaching, and twisting. It can also be expanded into recreational activities, such as swimming, tennis, golf, hiking, climbing, and other sports. Once we understand the client's desired activity, we can further evaluate what might be restricting their ability to perform that activity.

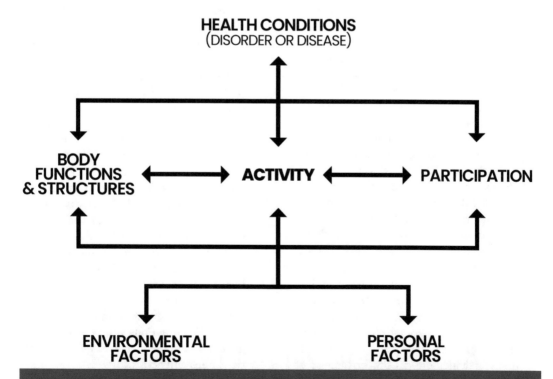

Figure 8-1. The World Health Organization's ICF model.

(Reproduced with permission from World Health Organization. Towards a common language for functioning, disability and health: ICF. Author; 2002:10. https://cdn.who.int/media/docs/default-source/classification/icf/icfbeginnersguide.pdf?sfvrsn =eead63d3_4&download=true)

- **Body Functions:** These are the physiological and psychological functions of body systems. These physical and psychological impairments are measurable and objective. These measures are often the objective measures found in a medical examination. In physical therapy, these measures may include range of motion, strength, girth, inflammation, reflexes, sensation, blood pressure, heart rate, endurance, and breath capacity.

- **Body Structures:** These consist of the anatomical parts of the body, including organs and systems. For the purposes of this book, structure includes the skeletal, myofascial, and nervous systems. In physical therapy, these are often measures of postural alignment, joint mobility and stability, soft tissue mobility and stability, nerve conduction, and motor reflexes.

- **Impairments:** These include problems in body function or structure representing a deficiency or variation from normal, usually leading to functional limitations. Structurally, a poorly aligned posture can potentially lead to limited range of motion of a joint, which could restrict normal movement and strength. Impairments are measurable and objective in nature. It is important to remember that not all impairments lead to functional or activity limitations. This classification process allows practitioners to prioritize interventions based on limitations caused by impairments that relate to participation. As mentioned earlier, this includes both psychological and physiological impairments.

- **Health Conditions:** These are disorders or diseases that influence the ability to participate in many of life's activities. A good example is something as common as osteoporosis. This condition restricts many activities due to the brittleness of bones and the risk of fracture. Metabolic, autoimmune, and cardiovascular disorders, like most pathologies, have their precautions and restrictions that influence one's ability to fully participate in their desired activities.

- **Environmental Factors:** These include the physical, social, and attitudinal environment in which people live and conduct their lives. Such factors as weather, work environment, lighting, workstations, stairs, slopes, and even assistance in the home by family members can influence one's ability to participate fully.

- **Personal Factors:** This refers to age, sex, ethnicity, socioeconomic status, belief models, self-efficacy, expectations, previous experiences, culture, values, and fears. This is the part of the ICF model that interests me the most. It is important to consider all the many factors that influence our well-being, as discussed earlier in this chapter, including but not limited to phenotypes of motor learning, individual biology, psychology, sensory interpretation, and much more.

- **Participation Restrictions:** These are problems an individual may experience with involvement in a life situation. The individual's limited access can be dependent on community or social access, or the lack thereof, rather than the individual's restrictions. An individual that requires a wheelchair for locomotion is only limited in this daily activity if there is a lack of wheelchair accessibility in the community. This also takes into consideration the societal demands the individual places on themselves. If an individual is involved in activities and roles that require greater function than another individual with theoretically the same impairment, then their limitations will be perceived as greater due to the increased demand from their roles and activities.

ASKING THE RIGHT QUESTIONS

All assessments must start with a few questions for the client. My mentor, Dr. Carol M. Davis, has been a great influence on my practice and has always placed the emphasis on practitioners engaging the client in the discovery of the answers. The premise that the client knows what they need, but they just do not know where to find it, has been a driving force to improve my interviewing skills and truly seek to understand my clients, what they need, and what they want.[12]

I have incorporated the following 3 interview questions that help me with the algorithm of the assessment:

1. What do you believe you should be able to participate in right now?
2. Do you believe you are currently able to participate in this activity at the level you desire?
3. If not, what do you believe is challenging or preventing you from participating at the level you desire?

These 3 questions can provide a plethora of information. The one thing I have learned is not to ever assume what the answer will be but to just listen to their answers. It is okay if the client struggles in their effort to articulate their answers. The answers many times might need further clarification by repeating back to the client what we heard and asking if this is a correct interpretation of what they believe and feel. It might take a few go-rounds before we have a clear agreement of what they believe (Box 8-1).

ASSESSMENT WITH PRINCIPLES OF MOVEMENT

In this final chapter, my intention is to provide guidelines on how the Principles of Movement can be used to assess our clients and design meaningful movement interventions. For many years, I have been testing algorithms to help understand the easiest way to achieve desired outcomes, especially for the young, less experienced practitioner. The algorithm is far from perfect, but it is my hope that it will be used as another tool in the practitioner's toolbox to better serve the individual.

After applying the ICF model to create a clear picture of what the client desires to participate in, we can ask the next question, which is if they can participate in that desired activity safely and efficiently. Once we define the movement and mental demands of the desired activity, we can select the movement tests from the Polestar Assessment Tool (PAT).

The PAT (see Appendix 8-1) was designed specifically for movement practitioners, such as mindful movement teachers, dance educators, martial artists, fitness instructors, and personal trainers who have not had formal training in medical or rehabilitative diagnostics. In teaching the PAT for more than 25 years, I have found that licensed professionals have appreciated the assessment tool in their practices. I can only hope that whether you are a doctor of rehabilitation or a dance teacher, you will find the following useful.

The PAT looks at alignment, mobility, control, and coordination throughout the body. Let us use an example of a client who wants to be able to coach their daughter's soccer team. The physical demands of the coach include being able to stand, walk, and run on the soccer field. It more than likely will require them to squat to the ground, bend over, and demonstrate multiplanar movements, such as teaching how to dribble the ball. We can now

BOX 8-1

A patient was referred to me for an evaluation and treatment for chronic neck pain. I asked him the 3 questions discussed before. He went on to relate to me that he is an auto mechanic and that he could not perform his work activities. He said that he had been to many therapists and chiropractors, but none were able to help him. When asked the third question (What prevents you from being able to work as an auto mechanic?), he responded, "I feel like my head is attached by a string and if I move my head the wrong way, my head will fall off." I repeated back what I heard him say, and for a moment, he looked at me as if I was crazy. He knew his neck was not attached by a string. I then asked him to place his hands around his neck and to observe the girth of his neck. Then I asked him to close his eyes and imagine assessing his neck as if it was an automobile in his garage. He then said, "It looks like the motor is seized up." I asked him how he would fix the motor. He responded, "I would break up some of the restrictions and lubricate the pistons." I then had him open his eyes, and I explained that this was my job, to remove restrictions, increase lubrication to the parts, and restore pain-free movement. I then asked him permission to treat his neck. After a couple successful treatment sessions, he returned to work. I realized that as long as he had the belief of his head being connected by a string, no therapist was going to have access to treating him. I also realized how important it is for the client to be able to tell their story.

choose 5 to 10 tests in the PAT to assess their status, including the half squat, full squat, goal post, marriage proposal lunge, Z-sit, push-up, and swan. These 7 tests can provide a lot of information regarding the client's ability to participate in their specific activity as a soccer coach. It is important to note, if the PAT does not have a test that correlates to their activity or is not sensitive enough, then we have the obligation to be creative and mimic the physical demands of the desired activity.

The principles can be used in a very systematic way to understand where movement deficiencies reside. I have created a diagram that depicts a strategy of how one might use the principles when assessing a functional movement task, such as squatting, sitting, walking, jumping, lifting, and so on (Figure 8-2).

The formula to grade the screening is based on a series of criteria within each test. These assessments are built on—you guessed it—the Principles of Movement. The sequence of each test is as follows. Can they perform the

test, for example, a full squat? If they perform the test with proper dynamic alignment and efficiency, then move on to the next test. If they do not, then continue down the algorithm. Each principle can influence the ability to successfully perform the task or test. In many cases, multiple principles can simultaneously impair movement and, more importantly, the quality of movement.

Many clients are unfamiliar with the different tests, and we do not always know if their inability to accurately complete the test is because it is new or they truly cannot achieve the movement or position. We often start with coordination by providing verbal, visual, or tactile cueing to improve the outcome of the test. If the client can make the correction from the cueing, then we can assume that the deficiency is probably due to their lack of experience, awareness, or coordination/movement integration. If the client cannot make the corrections with the practitioner's cueing, then continue down the algorithm to control mobility limitations.

The principle of control is often associated with load. To differentiate control limitations, we can modify the load by providing assistance during the half or full squat. If the client is able to perform the squat successfully with assistance, then we can assume that the limitation is partially due to lack of control and the program design will include a graded load strategy.

The principle of mobility is directly related to range of motion and distribution of movement. In the squat test, mobility is necessary in the ankle, knee, hip, lumbar, and thoracic spine. To differentiate mobility limitations, we can modify the range of motion. If we lift the client's heels up with a 2-inch (5-cm) lift and ask them to attempt the half squat again and they are able to perform the test with proper dynamic alignment, we can assume that the client was lacking mobility in ankle dorsiflexion. The intervention will include exercises and treatments to increase mobility in ankle dorsiflexion. The treatment or exercise plan might also include graded range of motion exercises so that the rest of the body can be conditioned with proper alignment and load. When the load is too great, we can modify the load either by eliminating gravity or by providing assistance. If providing assistance during the squat allows for successful dynamic alignment in the squat, then we can assume that control of the load was a factor and should be a focus in the intervention design.

The principle of breath is equally important and should be evaluated as well. It is not independent of any of the other principles and should be considered equally important. Breathing strategies can be incorporated into the principle of coordination. Verbal and tactile cueing to improve breath strategies can also improve the quality of movement. Improving breathing techniques can improve poor thorax and spine mobility associated with diminished breath capacity. Breath can also influence control. Intra-abdominal pressure (IAP) can improve or impair trunk control required with activities that increase load on

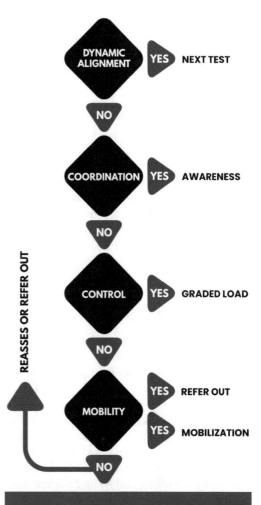

Figure 8-2. Polestar critical reasoning schematic.

the torso. My suggestion is to make sure that breathing is evaluated with every test. A couple good examples of the above are as follows:

- The lateral flexion test can be improved by providing directional cues to breathe into the convex side of the rib cage.

- Exhalation can significantly improve spine articulation in spine flexion, where holding one's breath (Valsalva) can impair mobility and distribution of movement.

- A controlled exhalation can greatly assist IAP when increasing load on a stable trunk.

The reality is that clients might have limitations on more than 1 principle, and some on all 5. In this case, I set a priority to address the Principles of Movement deficiencies in the following order: mobility, control (graded load), and coordination (movement integration). Although not a science, it helps me keep my strategy in place. By the end of the short assessment, I know what the client wants and where they are mentally and physically, and I know what is required to perform at their desired level of participation. I now have measurable outcomes that can inform the client and me of how the program is going and if our intervention is achieving the desired goals.

SAMPLE CASE

Marvin is a 67-year-old male client 6 months post–total anterolateral hip replacement. He has successfully completed all his therapy and is able to walk and perform most of his activities with no pain; he is very pleased with the surgery. Recently, his daughter and her family moved into town; they have 3 little children ranging in age from 18 months to 5 years old. His daughter and her husband are busy, as he describes, and he and his wife love to take care of their grandchildren as much as possible. He has one complaint, which is his inability to squat all the way to the floor to address the needs of his young grandchildren. He is coming to us to help him be able to get down on the ground and get back up. His surgeon says he has no physical or structural precautions secondary to the hip replacement, but per the patient, it has been more than 15 years since he has been able to get on the floor.

Some factors to consider in Marvin's case include his past physical activity. He was a collegiate American football player in his prime and continued with an active lifestyle of running, hiking, and working out in the gym until 10 years ago when his right hip restrictions ended most of his physical activity. He feels that he has a new lease on life because of the surgery. He has minimal medical concerns now other than high blood pressure, which is controlled with medication.

It is important to remember what Marvin wants from his intervention and what he believes is limiting his ability to get down and up from the floor to play with his grandkids. Historically, his limitation to getting up and down off the floor has been secondary to the chronic hip pain before hip surgery and a possible loss of mobility in the affected hip. Now he has a new hip with no medical limitations but still cannot get on the ground.

We know what activity he wants to be able to do so we can look at our PAT and select a few of the tests to assess his current movement status related to being able to get down and up from the ground. Another concern of his is the ability to sit on the ground for a short period of time to be with his grandkids. What tests would you choose?

The first tests that come to my mind are the half squat and the marriage proposal lunge. I would also like to see what his sitting tolerance is and would look at a long sit and a cross-legged position. In Marvin's case, he still might need to have a modification on the ground, such as a raised mat or low stool, so that he can tolerate sitting on the floor.

HALF SQUAT TEST

Marvin attempts to squat and gets about halfway down; he loses his alignment, his head goes forward, his back slouches, the lumbar spine flexes instead of his hips, and he must widen his legs. I also notice that he is holding his breath on the attempt.

MARRIAGE PROPOSAL LUNGE TEST

Marvin has trouble balancing. He shifts his front knee forward instead of flexing the front hip. He needs hand support to go half-way down and reports a big stretch in his back, thigh, and hip.

ASSESSMENT BY PRINCIPLE

BREATH

He is holding his breath, which will restrict spine movement. This tells me there is somewhere else he does not want to move, probably a habit to substitute for the lack of control in the trunk. This is a flag or place to make a note for your programming and teaching to remember to facilitate natural breathing in all planes first on its own and then with movement to optimize his movement efficiency.

ALIGNMENT

He loses the relationship between the head and thorax, the thorax and pelvis, and the lower extremities. He is given a series of verbal and tactile cues. If Marvin can successfully execute the tests with proper alignment after cueing, then we can attribute the deficiency to a lack of coordination.

COORDINATION

The loss of coordination could potentially be caused by years of compensation and habits to avoid flexing at the hip. If this is the case, then Marvin just needs to be re-educated in how to use his new hip and start building up the load tolerance. Move on to check out mobility and control.

MOBILITY

The loss of alignment could be caused by the loss of mobility in ankle dorsiflexion, hip adduction, flexion and internal rotation, or thoracic extension. Maybe lifting his heels up

on a half roll might take the load off the hip and back and allow Marvin to keep his axial elongation.

CONTROL

If it turns out that Marvin does have ample mobility, then he does not have proper control of the load of gravity needed to squat and lunge. Maybe he needs assistance or manipulation of gravity.

LOAD

Can Marvin do the squat or the lunge with assistance or in a foreign environment that diminishes the load and allows for a successful closed-chain movement through the full range of motion?

PLAN OF CARE USING THE PRINCIPLES OF MOVEMENT

In Marvin's case, the loss of alignment was caused by a combination of factors, but the most significant was the loss of mobility in his ankles and the lack of mobility into thoracic extension. Objectives for this treatment or exercise plan could start off as follows:

- Phase 1: Restoration of mobility, control, and breath
  - Increase ankle dorsiflexion
  - Increase standing tolerance
  - Increase thoracic extension
  - Increase breath mobility in all 3 planes

- Phase 2: Restoration of alignment and control
  - Emphasize alignment of the axial skeleton and lower extremities as tolerated
  - Gradually increase load during the squat and lunge activity, progressing from a foreign to a familiar environment

- Phase 3: Restore coordination
  - Practice many ways to get up and down off the ground
  - Celebrate successes along the way

This case study is oversimplified for demonstration purposes so that you can see the rationale and application. If there is a lack of mobility and control, then we work on that for a bit and gradually increase load, bring attention to alignment and breath, and practice until it is efficient and spontaneous. Marvin is now able to play with his grandkids without giving his hip a second thought!

CONCLUSION

It continues to be a great journey as we strive to improve our skills to provide the best care with the greatest outcomes. I mentioned early in the book my vision of a pathokinesiologist and a performance kinesiologist and how this professional title could represent everyone who desires to change the world through movement. As a movement practitioner, you fall into one or both categories. I love my profession and my ability to truly influence the lives of so many clients through the art and science of movement. Now it is your turn to see if the information in this book can help you in your assessment, design, facilitation, and achievement of desired movement objectives as a movement practitioner. I would love to hear how it is working for you, and I am always open to feedback to continue to improve our profession. Who knows? Maybe you will be helping me with the next edition of *Principles of Movement*. Until then, let us stay focused on the most important part of our profession, which is discovering the unique needs and designing unique movement programs to optimize the successful movement experience for our clients. Be happy!

OPEN-ENDED QUESTIONS

1 Conduct a practice interview with a colleague, and ask the subjective questions pertaining to "participation." How can you use this information to direct further objective testing and program design?

2 What dangers might occur as the practitioner if you assume what you see is what you get without having a detailed interview with the patient or client to assess what they believe and want for themselves?

3 Once you have defined what the client wants to participate in, describe what activities are needed to be performed safely to fully participate. How will you determine if they can do the associated activities safely?

4 Take a couple hours to practice the PAT with a colleague. Identify which tests might align better with specific activities. What PAT tests might be most applicable for someone who wants to play golf?

5 In your own words, how do the Principles of Movement refine the results of the PAT tests selected as part of the evaluation? How can you use them to identify the greatest deficits to address first?

OPEN-ENDED QUESTIONS

6 If a client can perform the test correctly with proper alignment after imagery tactile or verbal cueing, what assumption can you make regarding their exercise plan?

7 Explain in your own words what you would do next if a client could not correct their alignment during their squat tests with tactile and verbal cueing.

8 If alignment cannot be maintained during a test after awareness cueing or load modifications, where might you assume is the movement restriction? How would you differentiate between load modification and structural restrictions?

9 Discuss with a colleague how it might be possible for all 5 principles to be in deficit at the same time. How might you differentiate which principle to emphasize first?

10 Describe how you would use breath assessment in your evaluation. How might breath affect or not affect specific PAT tests? How would you measure the influence breath has on the quality of movement?

REFERENCES

1. van Dieën JH, Reeves NP, Kawchuk G, van Dillen LR, Hodges PW. Motor control changes in low back pain: divergence in presentations and mechanisms. *J Orthop Sports Phys Ther*. 2019;49(6):370-379.
2. Hides JA, Donelson R, Lee D, Prather H, Sahrmann SA, Hodges PW. Convergence and divergence of exercise-based approaches that incorporate motor control for the management of low back pain. *J Orthop Sports Phys Ther*. 2019;49(6):437-452.
3. Hodges PW, van Dieen JH, Cholewicki J. Time to reflect on the role of motor control in low back pain. *J Orthop Sports Phys Ther*. 2019;49(6):367-369.
4. Hodges PW, Danneels L. Changes in structure and function of the back muscles in low back pain: different time points, observations, and mechanisms. *J Orthop Sports Phys Ther*. 2019;49(6):464-476.
5. Hodges PW, Barbe MF, Loggia ML, Nijs J, Stone LS. Diverse role of biological plasticity in low back pain and its impact on sensorimotor control of the spine. *J Orthop Sports Phys Ther*. 2019;49(6):389-401.
6. Brumagne S, Diers M, Danneels L, Moseley GL, Hodges PW. Neuroplasticity of sensorimotor control in low back pain. *J Orthop Sports Phys Ther*. 2019;49(6):402-414.
7. Cholewicki J, Breen A, Popovich JM Jr, et al. Can biomechanics research lead to more effective treatment of low back pain? A point-counterpoint debate. *J Orthop Sports Phys Ther*. 2019;49(6):425-436.
8. Reeves NP, Cholewicki J, van Dieen JH, Kawchuk G, Hodges PW. Are stability and instability relevant concepts for back pain? *J Orthop Sports Phys Ther*. 2019;49(6):415-424.
9. Hodges PW. Hybrid approach to treatment tailoring for low back pain: a proposed model of care. *J Orthop Sports Phys Ther*. 2019;49(6):453-463.
10. van Dieën JH, Reeves NP, Kawchuk G, van Dillen LR, Hodges PW. Analysis of motor control in patients with low back pain: a key to personalized care? *J Orthop Sports Phys Ther*. 2019;49(6):380-388.
11. World Health Organization 2001. The International Classification of Functioning, Disability and Health (ICF). WHO. http://www.who.int/classifications/icf/en/
12. Davis CM. *Patient Practitioner Interaction: An Experiential Manual for Developing the Art of Health Care*. 5th ed. SLACK Incorporated; 2011.

APPENDIX 8-1

POLESTAR®

ASSESSMENT TOOL

PAT

GOAL POST

POLESTAR®
ASSESSMENT TOOL

SCORE _____ OUT OF **9** *points*

TESTS

The ability to stand in a neutral torso alignment • adequate thoracic mobility to align back of head, ribs, and pelvis. The ability to stand in a neutral torso alignment • adequate thoracic mobility to align back of head, ribs, and pelvis.

Shoulder girdle mobility into abduction and external rotation *(soft tissue and shoulder joint)* in Position 1

Shoulder girdle mobility into upward rotation, abduction, and flexion *(soft tissue and shoulder joint)* in Position 2

Torso control during Positions 1 and 2

If needed, test each side independently

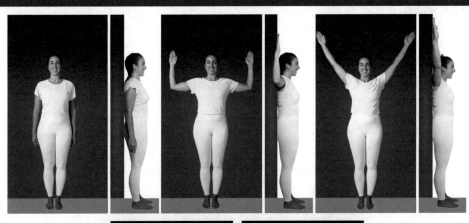

FAULTY EXECUTION

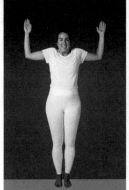
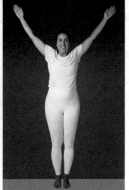

SHOULDERS ELEVATED

GOAL POST
continuation

POLESTAR®
ASSESSMENT TOOL

START POSITION
Stand against wall with back of head, mid-thoracic, buttocks touching wall, without ribs jutting foward. Heels 2"/5cm from wall. Gaze forward.

☐ 1 = Stand with head, mid-thorax, and pelvis touching wall, without ribs jutting forward

☐ 1 = Gaze horizontal

☐ 1 = Relaxed in position, no excessive tension in the cervical spine or ribs

▶ Needed cueing to accomplish the test: _____

▶ Needed modification to accomplish the test: _____

▶ List reason for modification: _____

▶ What prevented full and comfortable execution of the test: _____

ARM POSITION 1
Able to touch back of arm, wrist and hand against the wall in goal post position and:

☐ 1 = Maintain head, mid-thoracic, and rib cage position without ribs jutting forward

☐ 1 = Maintain pelvis position and spine position

☐ 1 = Maintain scapular position without elevation, adduction, or UT over-recruitment

▶ Needed cueing to accomplish the test: _____

▶ Needed modification to accomplish the test: _____

▶ List reason for modification: _____

▶ What prevented full and comfortable execution of the test: _____

ARM POSITION 2
Able to touch back of arm, wrist and hand against the wall in goal post position and:

☐ 1 = Maintain head, mid-thoracic, and rib cage position without ribs jutting forward

☐ 1 = Maintain pelvis position and spine position

☐ 1 = Maintain scapular position without elevation, adduction, or UT over-recruitment

▶ Needed cueing to accomplish the test: _____

▶ Needed modification to accomplish the test: _____

▶ List reason for modification: _____

▶ What prevented full and comfortable execution of the test: _____

FULL SQUAT

POLESTAR®
ASSESSMENT TOOL

SCORE _____ **OUT OF** **8** *points* FOR EACH TEST

TESTS　　　Ability to perform a full squat with either heels up or heels down

FULL SQUAT HEELS UP:
Lower extremity strength, mobility, alignment, control, and balance.

Keep torso vertical and heels down, flex hips, knees, and ankles as far as possible.
Pause, continue to descend allowing heels to rise, moving into full knee flexion.
Return to standing. Maintain neutral spine and vertical torso throughout the movement.

☐ 1 = Able to bend knees (half squat) to at least 75 degrees with heels down, torso vertical, and neutral spine

☐ 1 = Keeps lower extremity alignment, avoiding pronation and valgus

☐ 1 = Keeps pelvis neutral, minimizing an anterior or posterior tilt

☐ 1 = Keeps rib cage aligned over pelvis, avoiding shifting of ribs forward

☐ 1 = Keeps torso vertical

☐ 1 = Keeps head in alignment, avoiding jutting chin or head forward

☐ 1 = Keeps shoulder girdle organized, avoiding elevation or protraction

☐ 1 = Able to descend into full knee flexion (full squat)

▶ Needed cueing to accomplish the test. _____

▶ Needed modification to accomplish the test: _____

▶ List reason for modification: _____

▶ What prevented full and comfortable execution of the test: _____

Heels up can be used when squatting to lift something heavy to maintain a more neutral spine position.

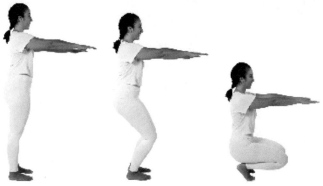

FULL SQUAT
continuation

POLESTAR®
ASSESSMENT TOOL

FULL SQUAT HEELS DOWN:
Lower extremity strength, mobility, alignment, control, and balance.

Keep torso vertical and heels down, flex hips, knees, and ankles as far as possible. Pause, continue to descend until hips and knees are in full flexion. Return to standing. Maintain vertical torso throughout the movement.

- ☐ 1 = Able to bend knees (half squat) to at least 75 degrees with heels down, torso vertical, and neutral spine
- ☐ 1 = Keeps lower extremity alignment, avoiding pronation and valgus
- ☐ 1 = Keeps rib cage aligned over pelvis, avoiding shifting of ribs forward
- ☐ 1 = Keeps torso vertical
- ☐ 1 = Keeps head in alignment, avoiding jutting chin or head forward
- ☐ 1 = Keeps shoulder girdle organized, avoiding elevation or protraction
- ☐ 1 = Able to lengthen lumbar spine in full squat position
- ☐ 1 = Able to descend into full knee flexion (full squat)

▶ Needed cueing to accomplish the test: _____

▶ Needed modification to accomplish the test: _____

▶ List reason for modification: _____

▶ What prevented full and comfortable execution of the test: _____

Heels down is often used more for work or recreation that takes place on the ground.

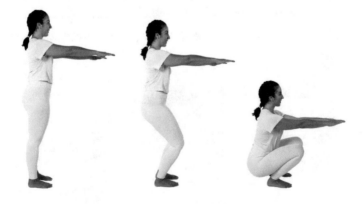

FULL SQUAT
continuation

POLESTAR®
ASSESSMENT TOOL

FAULTY EXECUTION

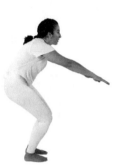

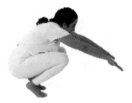
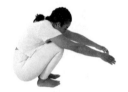

SPINE FLEXION   SPINE FLEXION   SPINE FLEXION
                                                                 WEIGHT BACK ON HEELS
                                                                 POSSIBLE LACK OF DORSIFLEXION

MARRIAGE PROPOSAL

POLESTAR®
ASSESSMENT TOOL

SCORE _____ **OUT OF** **8** *points*

TESTS	Leg strength and balance in narrow staggered stance	Hip flexion mobility *(hip disassociation in front hip)*	Hip adductor mobility in narrow stance	Hip neutral mobility & control in back leg

Keep torso vertical, and parallel lower extremity alignment, step right foot at least 36"/90cm forward if subject is between 5-6'/150-180cm tall and at least 40"/100cm forward if subject is over 6'/180cm tall. (Measure from toes of right foot to toes of left foot). Feet 3-4"/7-10cm apart side to side. Bend both knees and begin to descend toward the floor without torso or weight shifting forward. Front tibia and back femur should be vertical at bottom of lunge. Maintain neutral pelvis and vertical torso throughout the movement.

Subject may wear shoes for the Lunge Test if great toe dorsiflexion is limited/painful or ball of foot is sensitive on the floor.

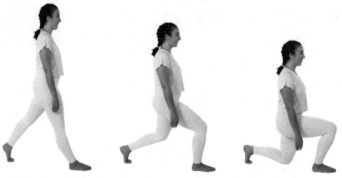

R **L**

- [ ] .5 [ ] .5 = Maintain lower extremity alignment with equal knee flexion bilaterally, keeping front tibia vertical
- [ ] .5 [ ] .5 = Keeps pelvis neutral in all planes
- [ ] .5 [ ] .5 = Keeps rib cage centered over pelvis, avoiding lower ribs shifting forward or back
- [ ] .5 [ ] .5 = Keeps torso vertical
- [ ] .5 [ ] .5 = Keeps head in alignment, avoiding forward head or jutting chin
- [ ] .5 [ ] .5 = Keeps shoulder girdle organized, avoiding protraction or elevation
- [ ] 1 [ ] 1 = Bend knees so that back knee touches the floor and rise up again maintaining pelvis level, neutral spine, and torso vertical

▶ Needed cueing to accomplish the test: _____

▶ Needed modification to accomplish the test: _____

▶ List reason for modification: _____

▶ What prevented full and comfortable execution of the test: _____

MARRIAGE PROPOSAL

continuation

POLESTAR®
ASSESSMENT TOOL

FAULTY EXECUTION

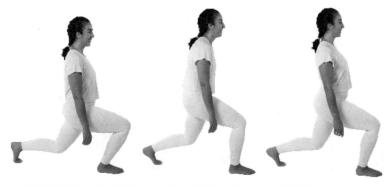

WEIGHT SHIFTED FORWARD   SPINE IN FLEXION   SPINE IN EXTENSION

FAULTY EXECUTION

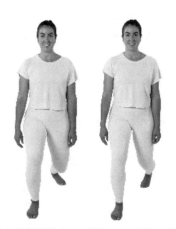

BACK ANKLE PRONATED OR SUPINATED

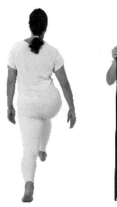

HIP HIKE

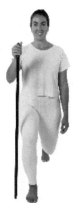

WITH ASSISTANCE

Z•SIT

POLESTAR®
ASSESSMENT TOOL

SCORE _____ OUT OF **4** *points*

TESTS	Seated hip internal and external rotation ROM in 90* of hip flexion

Sit with legs swept to one side.
Put feet in comfortable position.
Subject should be able to easily sit in position with spine in neutral.

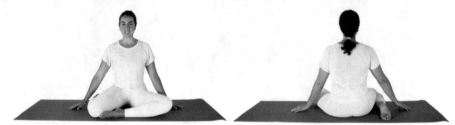

R   **L**

- ☐ .5 ☐ .5 =   Neutral pelvis in sagittal plane (no anterior or posterior tilt of the pelvis)
- ☐ .5 ☐ .5 =   Vertical, neutral spine (no lateral shift or sidebending)
- ☐ .5 ☐ .5 =   Iliac height fairly level and rib to pelvis distance fairly equal
- ☐ .5 ☐ .5 =   Relaxed in position (subject able to sit easily for several minutes)

▶ Needed cueing to accomplish the test: _____

▶ Needed modification to accomplish the test: _____

▶ List reason for modification: _____

▶ What prevented full and comfortable execution of the test: _____

FAULTY EXECUTION

SIDEBENDING   HAND SUPPORT   POOR POSTURE

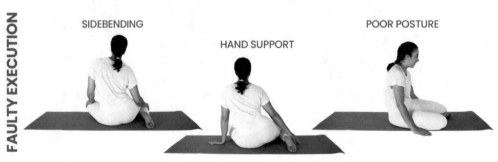

SWAN

POLESTAR®
ASSESSMENT TOOL

SCORE _____ OUT OF **17** *points*

TESTS	Thoracic spine extension mobility	Ability to attain thoracic and hip extension in a curved shape	Torso and pelvic control

CERVICAL AND UPPER THORACIC MOVEMENT AND CONTROL

Lie prone, neutral spine and pelvis, forehead on hands.
Lift head from hands and move upper thoracic spine into extension.
Maintain the position of the body and lift arms from mat, hands to forehead.
Legs stay on the mat. Eye gaze stays toward backs of hands.

Able to maintain lower torso and pelvic position and:

☐ 1 = Extend cervical spine
☐ 1 = Extend upper thoracic spine
☐ 1 = Extend upper thoracic spine without scapular protraction or elevation
☐ 1 = Extend upper thoracic spine without changing lumbo-pelvic position
☐ 1 = Lift forearms off the mat back of hands to touch forehead

▶ Needed cueing to accomplish the test: _____
▶ Needed modification to accomplish the test: _____
▶ List reason for modification: _____
▶ What prevented full and comfortable execution of the test: _____

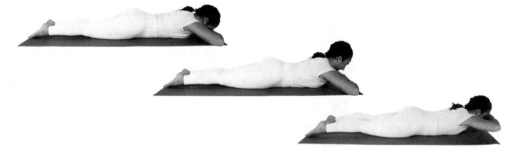

Transition: Maintain thoracic extension and place the arms on the mat in the goal post position

SWAN
continuation

MID THORACIC MOVEMENT AND CONTROL

Able to maintain head and torso position and:

- [ ] 1 = Extend mid-thoracic spine
- [ ] 1 = Extend mid-thoracic spine without scapular protraction or elevation
- [ ] 1 = Extend mid-thoracic spine without increasing cervical or lumbar extension
- [ ] 1 = Lift forearms off the mat in goal post position without scapular elevation

▶ Needed cueing to accomplish the test: _____

▶ Needed modification to accomplish the test: _____

▶ List reason for modification: _____

▶ What prevented full and comfortable execution of the test: _____

Transition: Maintain thoracic extension and place the hands on the mat near the lower ribs

LOWER THORACIC MOVEMENT AND CONTROL

Maintain thoracic extension and place the hands on the mat near the lower ribs

- [ ] 1 = Extend lower thoracic spine
- [ ] 1 = Extend lower thoracic spine without changing scapular position
- [ ] 1 = Extend lower thoracic spine without increasing cervical or lumbar extension
- [ ] 1 = Lift hands off the mat at least 1"

▶ Needed cueing to accomplish the test: _____

▶ Needed modification to accomplish the test: _____

▶ List reason for modification: _____

▶ What prevented full and comfortable execution of the test: _____

Transition: Place hands on the mat and press into full swan with hands under shoulders

SWAN

continuation

POLESTAR®
ASSESSMENT TOOL

FULL SWAN

☐ 1 = Able to extend the arms with the heels of the hands under the shoulders

☐ 1 = Able to straighten arms without locking elbows or changing scapular position

☐ 1 = Able to straighten arms without ribs jutting forward

☐ 1 = Able to straighten arms and extend hips without increasing lumbar extension

▶ Needed cueing to accomplish the test: _____

▶ Needed modification to accomplish the test: _____

▶ List reason for modification: _____

▶ What prevented full and comfortable execution of the test: _____

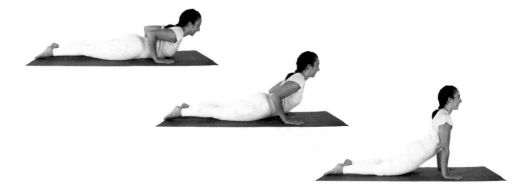

FAULTY EXECUTION

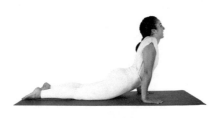

ELBOWS LOCKED, SCAPULA ELEVATED

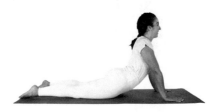

LUMBAR EXTENSION
HANDS FORWARD OF SHOULDERS

FOR ADDITIONAL RESOURCES,
INCLUDING THE FULL
POLESTAR ASSESSMENT TOOL

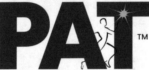

USE THIS QR CODE

INDEX

Printed in the United States
by Baker & Taylor Publisher Services